Handbook on
Clinical Approach to Respiratory Medicine

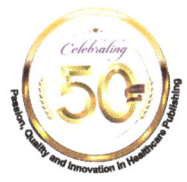

Handbook on
Clinical Approach to Respiratory Medicine

SECOND EDITION

K Surendra Menon MD
Former Professor and Head
Department of Pulmonary Medicine
Medical Education Service
Government of Kerala
Kerala, India

R Pajanivel MD FRCP
Professor and Head
Department of Pulmonary Medicine
Mahatma Gandhi Medical College and Research Institute
Sri Balaji Vidyapeeth
Puducherry, India

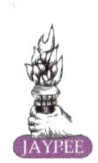

JAYPEE BROTHERS MEDICAL PUBLISHERS
The Health Sciences Publisher
New Delhi | London

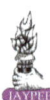 **Jaypee Brothers Medical Publishers (P) Ltd**

Headquarters
Jaypee Brothers Medical Publishers (P) Ltd
4838/24, Ansari Road, Daryaganj
New Delhi 110 002, India
Phone: +91-11-43574357
Fax: +91-11-43574314
Email: jaypee@jaypeebrothers.com

Overseas Offices
J.P. Medical Ltd
83 Victoria Street, London
SW1H 0HW (UK)
Phone: +44 20 3170 8910
Fax: +44 (0)20 3008 6180
Email: info@jpmedpub.com

Website: www.jaypeebrothers.com
Website: www.jaypeedigital.com

© 2021, Jaypee Brothers Medical Publishers

The views and opinions expressed in this book are solely those of the original contributor(s)/author(s) and do not necessarily represent those of editor(s) of the book.

All rights reserved. No part of this publication may be reproduced, stored or transmitted in any form or by any means, electronic, mechanical, photocopying, recording or otherwise, without the prior permission in writing of the publishers.

All brand names and product names used in this book are trade names, service marks, trademarks or registered trademarks of their respective owners. The publisher is not associated with any product or vendor mentioned in this book.

Medical knowledge and practice change constantly. This book is designed to provide accurate, authoritative information about the subject matter in question. However, readers are advised to check the most current information available on procedures included and check information from the manufacturer of each product to be administered, to verify the recommended dose, formula, method and duration of administration, adverse effects and contraindications. It is the responsibility of the practitioner to take all appropriate safety precautions. Neither the publisher nor the author(s)/editor(s) assume any liability for any injury and/or damage to persons or property arising from or related to use of material in this book.

This book is sold on the understanding that the publisher is not engaged in providing professional medical services. If such advice or services are required, the services of a competent medical professional should be sought.

Every effort has been made where necessary to contact holders of copyright to obtain permission to reproduce copyright material. If any have been inadvertently overlooked, the publisher will be pleased to make the necessary arrangements at the first opportunity. The **CD/DVD-ROM** (if any) provided in the sealed envelope with this book is complimentary and free of cost. **Not meant for sale**.

Inquiries for bulk sales may be solicited at: jaypee@jaypeebrothers.com

Handbook on Clinical Approach to Respiratory Medicine / K Surendra Menon, R Pajanivel
First Edition: 2017
Second Edition: **2021**

ISBN: 978-93-90595-73-0

Printed at

Dedicated To

Our second edition is dedicated to
The Health Professionals
who are fighting coronavirus disease 2019 (COVID-19)
day in and day out.

Preface to the Second Edition

Handbook On Clinical Approach to Respiratory Medicine is published with the intention of reaching out to the undergraduates, interns, and postgraduates to understand the importance of proper case taking. The authors are happy that this book is well-received and appreciated. This gives us the extra drive to publish the second edition with the addition of chapters like "Interpreting Chest X-rays in a Systematic Way" which is well-illustrated for better understanding and a list of frequently asked questions in clinical examination and viva.

Medicine is all about knowledge and observation. The essential element is the decisional process by probing history, recognition of signs, and clinical reasoning. Hands, ears, and the brain play a major part in diagnosing in spite of the laboratory tools available. As scientists, we are on a mission to alleviate the patients' suffering and have to go deeper into every aspect of the patient's disease process.

The art of history taking and proper examination of the patient is almost becoming extinct. This book confines basically to case taking in respiratory medicine and will give the reader a deeper insight into history taking and examination of the patient. This methodology will help in examining the other systems such as cardiovascular system (CVS), central nervous system (CNS), etc. Without a correct diagnosis, all efforts will be futile to treat the patient.

K Surendra Menon
R Pajanivel

Preface to the First Edition

Handbook on Clinical Approach to Respiratory Medicine is published with the intention of reaching out to the undergraduates, interns and postgraduates to understand the importance of proper case taking. Medicine is all about knowledge and observation. The essential element is the decisional process by probing history, recognition of signs and clinical reasoning. Hands, ears and the brain play a major role in diagnosing in spite of the laboratory tools available. As scientists, we are on a mission to alleviate the patients' sufferings and have to go deeper into every aspect of the patient's disease process.

The art of history taking and proper examination of the patient has become almost extinct. This book confines basically to case taking in respiratory medicine and will give the reader a deeper insight into history taking and examination of the patient. This methodology will help the reader in examining the other systems like CVS, CNS, etc. Without a correct diagnosis, all our efforts will be futile to treat the patient.

K Surendra Menon
R Pajanivel

Acknowledgments

We express our gratitude to our family members, all the faculty, and postgraduate students of the department. It is imperative to thank all the health professionals including our old students who are actively involved in this fight against the coronavirus all over the world.

Contents

1. **Anatomical Principles** — 1
   Important Anatomical Landmarks 1

2. **Symptomatology** — 17
   Cardinal Rule to History Taking 17
   Symptoms of Respiratory Diseases 19
   History Taking 32
   Making Provisional Diagnosis from History Obtained 34

3. **Examination of Respiratory System** — 37
   Vital Signs 37
   General Physical Examination 38
   Examination of Respiratory System 47

4. **Common Investigations in Respiratory Evaluation** — 81
   Diagnostic Tests 81
   Certain Important Tests (Not Commonly Done) 84

5. **Roentgenography: "A Step-by-step Approach to Reading of Chest X-ray"** — 89
   Posteroanterior View 90
   Anteroposterior View 91
   Lateral View of X-ray (Right Lateral and Left Lateral) 91
   Lateral Decubitus View 93
   Lordotic View 93
   Oblique View 95
   Common Terms 95
   Systematic Reading of Chest X-ray 96
   Pitfalls of Chest X-ray Interpretation 121
   Reading Chest X-rays: Tips 122

6. **Management of Pulmonary Emergencies** 123
   Acute Exacerbation of Bronchial Asthma 123
   Acute Exacerbation of Chronic Obstructive
   Pulmonary Disease 130
   Tension Pneumothorax 132
   Hemoptysis 134
   Respiratory Failure 136

7. **Viva Voce Questions and Bedside Questions** 139
   Viva Voce Questions 139
   Clinical Examination Questions 145

   Index **149**

Introduction

The content of the book emphasizes on the correct way of history taking, examination of the patient, relevant investigations, and arriving at a final diagnosis.

History taking is the time the doctor and the patient get to know each other and the patients' fears and concerns can be understood. The skills in taking history develop with experience, so students are encouraged to take history independently. Difficult diagnostic problems are more often solved by carefully taken history than by a battery of laboratory tests. At the end of history taking, we may be able to come to a few differential diagnoses before touching the patient. Our studies have shown that the correct history taking will make us zero in, onto a possible diagnosis in most of the cases, i.e., about 80%.

All systems are also required to be examined. As an examinee, quick history taking without missing any relevant points is essential and the last minute panic can be avoided, especially while appearing for the examination. It is advisable to finish the history taking in 10–12 minutes. But remember, this pattern has to be followed after graduation also to become a successful clinician.

Symptoms narrated by the patient should be carefully listened to and as a "medical detective" pertinent questions should be asked as some patients may go off the track. Patient's complaints should be documented and analyzed. Like a perfect diplomat, we should show tactfulness and patience when the subject mentions the complaint.

In the second edition, we are adding two chapters: X-ray of Chest and Commonly Asked Clinical Examination and Viva Voce Questions. The questions cover all the aspects of pulmonary medicine.

All the diagrams and photos are schematic (not to scale).

CHAPTER 1

Anatomical Principles

IMPORTANT ANATOMICAL LANDMARKS

One should have a clear understanding of anatomy of the respiratory system to perform a proper physical examination. Some of the important anatomical landmarks are outlined below.

The upper respiratory tract starts from the mouth or nose and includes all the structures in the mouth, nose, and sinus up to the larynx (the details of which will be discussed later). Lower respiratory tract starts from the lower border of cricoid cartilage which includes the trachea, airways, and lung parenchyma containing alveoli.

Trachea

- Starts from cricoid cartilage (lower border of larynx at the level of 6th cervical vertebra posteriorly) to sternal angle anteriorly (angle of Louis) and T5 spinous process posteriorly, where it divides into left and right main stem bronchi. The inner diameter is 25 mm and the length is about 10-16 cm.
- Trachea is generally in the midline, but slight deviation to right may occur in normal individuals (by right aortic arch

and weight of right lung). The weight of right adult lung ranges from 375 to 550 g and the left lung ranges from 325 to 450 g.
- Trachea has intra- and extrathoracic components. This has important bearing in the understanding of physiology of variable obstruction.

The spinous process is an important landmark because of its prominence and thoracic spines can be counted below it.

Angle of Louis

- Angle of Louis is the angle between the body of sternum and manubrium. Many important landmarks occur at this level:
    - 2nd rib articulates with manubrium sterni at this site. The ribs are counted anteriorly starting from this point.
    - Carina of trachea is at this level and it branches into right and left bronchi.
    - Mediastinum is divided into superior and inferior at this level.

With the help of surface anatomy, the thorax is arbitrarily divided into various spaces and lines. Description of abnormal signs in relation to the ribs, intercostal spaces (areas), and lines help to localize the lesion anatomically (upper lobe, lower lobe, middle lobe, etc.).

It is a significant anatomical landmarks as:
- Ribs are counted from this level to downward. 2nd rib lies at sternal angle.
- It marks the plane of separation of superior and inferior mediastinum.
- Ascending aorta ends, arch of aorta starts and ends, and descending aorta begins at this level.
- Trachea divides into two principle bronchi (right and left).

- Azygos vein arches over the roof of the right lung and opens in superior vena cava (SVC).
- Pulmonary trunk divides into two pulmonary arteries below this level.
- Thoracic duct crosses from right to left side and reaches left side at the level of sternal angle.
- It marks the upper limit of the base of the heart.
- Cardiac plexus are situated at the same level.

Ribs

Anteriorly ribs are counted down starting from 2nd rib. There are 12 ribs and 11 interspaces in each hemithorax. You can also count up from 12th rib. Inferior angle of scapula overlies 7th thoracic rib posteriorly.

Spaces/Areas (Chest Topography)

Anteriorly, the spaces are supraclavicular, infraclavicular and mammary, and Traube's space (**Fig. 1**).

- *Supraclavicular*: Space above clavicle.
- *Infraclavicular*: Space below clavicle up to 2nd intercostal space.
- *Mammary*: Space below infraclavicular area, i.e., 2nd to 6th intercostal space
- *Traube's (semilunar) space*: It is a crescent-shaped space, encompassed by the lower border of the left lung, the anterior border of the spleen, the left costal margin, and the inferior margin of the left lobe of the liver. Thus, its surface markings are respectively the left 6th rib superiorly, the left anterior axillary line laterally, and the left costal margin inferiorly. In other words, left 6th rib in the midclavicular line to 8th costal cartilage in the parasternal line, then along the left costal margin to the

4 | Anatomical Principles

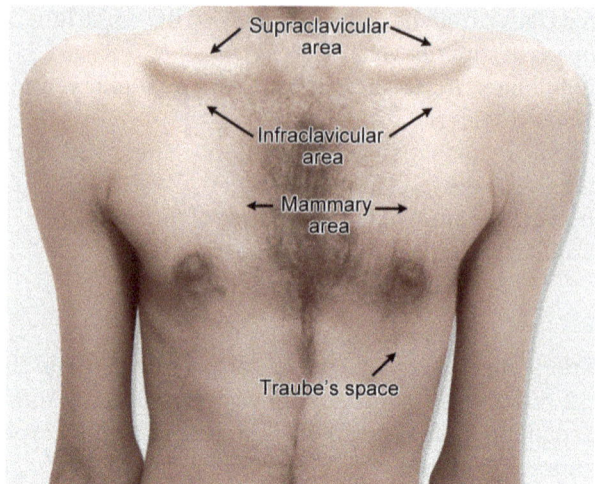

FIG. 1: Chest topography—space/area.

11th rib in the midaxillary line and then the 9th rib in midaxillary line.

Laterally, the spaces are axillary and infra-axillary spaces bound in between by two axillary folds. Anterior axillary fold is formed by pectoralis major muscle and posterior axillary fold by latissimus dorsi and teres major muscles.

- *Axillary area*: Space up to 5th intercostal space in midaxillary line (on the right where the horizontal fissure meets the oblique fissure).
- *Infra-axillary area*: Below the 5th intercostal space to 7th intercostal space.

Posteriorly, the spaces are suprascapular, interscapular, and infrascapular spaces (**Fig. 2**).

- *Suprascapular area*: From the apex to the spine of scapula.
- *Interscapular area*: From the spine of scapula to the angle of scapula.

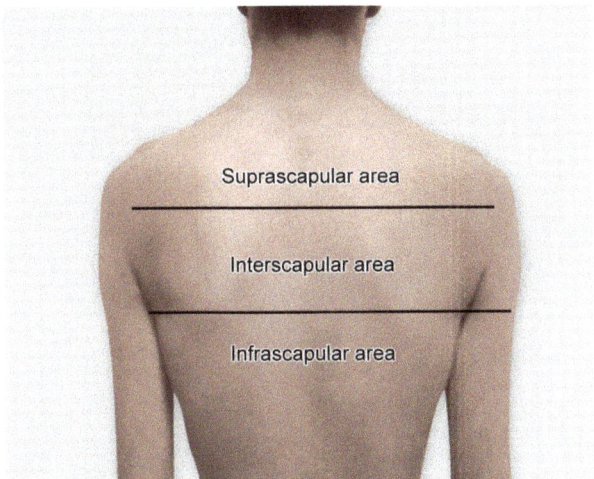

FIG. 2: Posterior spaces.

- *Infrascapular area*: From the angle of scapula to the 11th rib.

Lines

Following are the imaginary vertical lines in the chest: Midsternal, parasternal, midclavicular, anterior axillary, midaxillary, posterior axillary, infrascapular, and vertebral lines (**Figs. 3** to **5**).

- *Midsternal line*: A vertical line down the middle of sternum.
- *Parasternal line*: A vertical line along lateral edges of sternum.
- *Midclavicular line*: A vertical line from midpoint of clavicle.
- *Anterior axillary line*: A vertical line along anterior axillary fold.

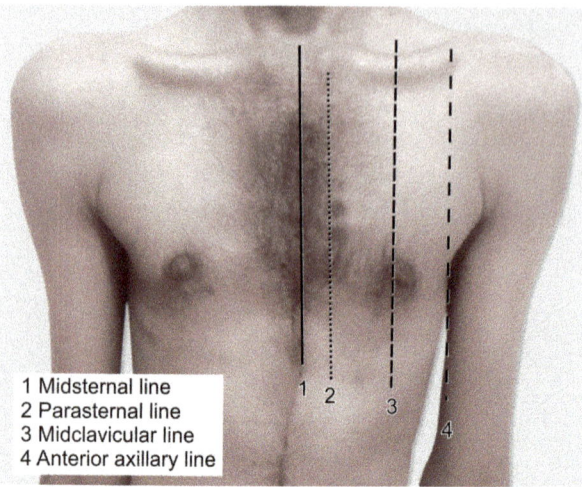

FIG. 3: Chest topography—important lines on anterior chest wall.

1 Midsternal line
2 Parasternal line
3 Midclavicular line
4 Anterior axillary line

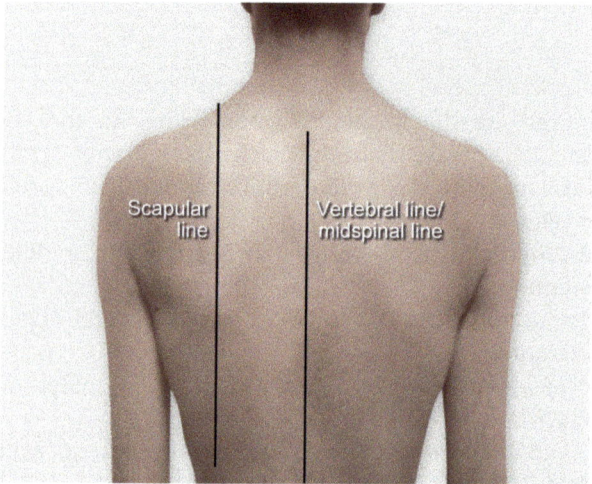

FIG. 4: Important lines on posterior chest wall.

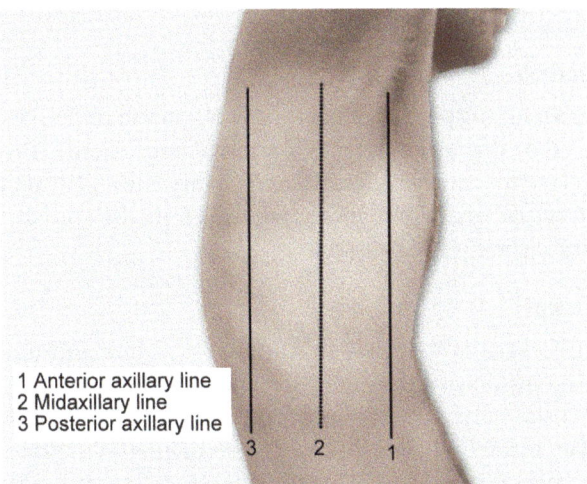

FIG. 5: Important lines on lateral chest wall.

1 Anterior axillary line
2 Midaxillary line
3 Posterior axillary line

- *Midaxillary line*: A vertical line at midpoint between anterior and posterior axillary line. There is less muscle attachment here, so it is the ideal place for putting intercostal drain and for thoracoscopy incision. This is also called *safe triangle* because there is less risk of injuring blood vessels like internal mammary artery and damage to muscle and breast tissue.
  - *Safe triangle*: It is bordered by the anterior border of the latissimus dorsi, the lateral border of the pectoralis major muscle, inferiorly by horizontal line from the nipple (5th intercostals space) just above the rib (to avoid neurovascular bundle) and superiorly by the axilla.
- *Posterior axillary line*: Along posterior axillary fold.
- *Scapular line*: Starting from the suprascapular area passing down the inferior angle of scapula.
- *Vertebral line*: Over spinous processes in the midline.

Surface Anatomy of Lungs

Right Lung

With a marking pen, start 3 cm above clavicle in midclavicular line, come down along right parasternal line, to join 6th rib in midclavicular line, to 8th rib in midaxillary line and to 10th rib posteriorly. Posterior marking of lung is from the apex to 10th thoracic vertebra posteriorly.

Left Lung

Start 3 cm above clavicle in midclavicular line and draw a line going downward along the parasternal margin up to 4th costal cartilage. Between 4th and 6th costal cartilage, deviate to left by 4 cm. The lower levels of lung—6th rib in the midclavicular line, 8th rib in the midaxillary line, and 10th rib in the scapular line.

Kronig's Isthmus

It is an area about 5-7 cm in the supraclavicular region. It is bound medially by scalenus muscle, laterally by acromion process of scapula, anteriorly by clavicle, and posteriorly by trapezius muscle.

Clinical Significance

Normal percussion over Kronig's isthmus is resonant. The percussion note becomes hyperresonant in emphysema and impaired in early tuberculosis and apical lung tumors.

Surface Anatomy of Lobes (Figs. 6 to 8)

Oblique fissure extends on the left from the tip of spinous process of the T3 vertebra that extends down to the level of 6th costochondral junction anteriorly. In taking this route, the approximate path of the 6th rib is followed. The posterior

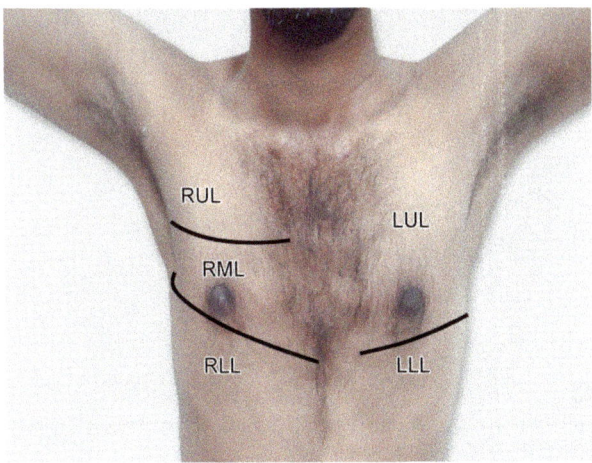

(LLL: left lower lobe; LUL: left upper lobe; RLL: right lower lobe; RML: right middle lobe; RUL: right upper lobe)

FIG. 6: Anterior surface markings of the lung lobes.

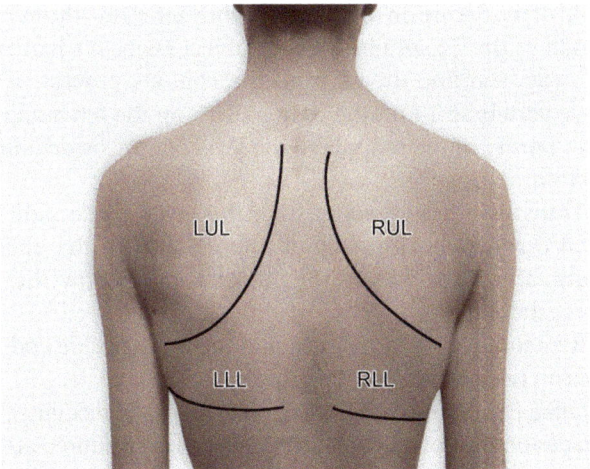

(LLL: left lower lobe; LUL: left upper lobe; RLL: right lower lobe; RUL: right upper lobe)

FIG. 7: Posterior surface markings of the lung lobes.

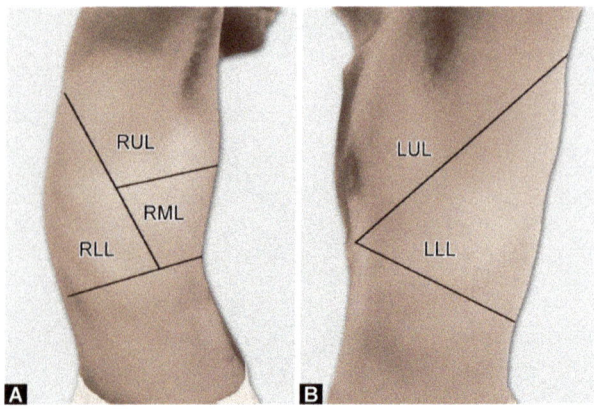

(LLL: left lower lobe; LUL: left upper lobe; RLL: right lower lobe; RML: right middle lobe; RUL: right upper lobe)

FIGS. 8A AND B: Lateral surface markings of the lung lobes. (A) Right lung; and (B) Left lung.

origin of the fissure on the right is slightly inferior—the inferior margin of the T4 vertebra. If the subject keeps his hands on the head, the line drawn from the spinous process of the above vertebrae T4 on the right and T3 on the left along the lower border of the scapula to the level of 6th costochondral junction.

Transverse fissure starts from the level of the right 4th costal cartilage horizontally to a junction with the oblique fissure at approximately the midaxillary line in the 5th intercostal space.

Remember there are three lobes on the right side and two lobes on the left side normally.

Once the fissures are drawn, one can easily recognize the surface anatomy of lobes of lungs. One can then appreciate the importance of examining the patient in all anatomical areas mentioned above to identify the lobes. Most of the lower lobe is in back, the upper lobe is in front, and the middle lobe is in front and in the axilla all the three (right) lobes are present.

Bronchopulmonary Segments

It is a wedge of lung tissue supplied by a single bronchus and corresponding pulmonary artery and vein. There are ten segments in right lung and eight segments in left lung (**Table 1**).

Muscles of Respiration

There are two types of muscles of respiration—principal and accessory muscles.

TABLE 1: Bronchopulmonary segments.

Right lung	Left lung
Right upper lobe bronchus	**Left upper lobe bronchus**
• Apical segment (1)	• Apicoposterior segment (1 and 2)
• Posterior segment (2)	• Anterior segment (3)
• Anterior segment (3)	–
Right middle lobe bronchus	**Lingula**
• Lateral segment (4)	• Superior segment (4)
• Medial segment (5)	• Inferior segment (5)
• Apical (superior) segment (6)	• Apical (6)
• Medial basal segment (7)	–
• Anterior basal segment (8)	• Anterior basal segment (8)
• Lateral basal segment (9)	• Lateral basal (9)
• Posterior basal segment (10)	• Posterior basal (10)

Note: No medial basal segment in left lung.

Principal muscles are used during normal inspiration while accessory muscles are used during forced breathing (heavy exercise and exacerbations of obstructive airway diseases).

Principal muscles include external intercostals, interchondral part of internal intercostals, and diaphragm.

The width of the thoracic cavity (lateral and anteroposterior diameter) is increased by external and interchondral part of internal intercostals which elevate the ribs. The lateral dimensions of the thorax are increased by the bucket handle movement of the ribs. Diaphragm contracts to increase the vertical dimensions of thoracic cavity and also aids in elevation of lower ribs and abdominal contents are pushed downward. *Accessory muscles* of inspiration are sternocleidomastoid which elevates the sternum and scalene muscles (anterior, middle, and posterior) elevate the first two ribs.

Remember to look for alae nasi when the patient is in respiratory distress that means a fall in forced expiratory volume in the first second (FEV_1) by 30%.

Muscles of expiration: It is passive as no muscle involvement in normal breathing. The process is simply done by elastic recoil of the lungs and the rib cage.

But during active breathing (exercise), the interchondral part of the internal intercostal muscles assists in active expiration by pulling the ribs downward and inward. They also prevent bulging of intercostal spaces during straining such as vigorous coughing and vomiting. The abdominal muscles when contract (rectus abdominis, external oblique, internal oblique, and transversus abdominis), intra-abdominal pressure increases and push the diaphragm upward and force the air out of the lungs.

Diaphragm (Fig. 9)

The diaphragm is a dome-shaped structure containing muscle and fibrous tissue that separates the thoracic cavity from the abdomen. The dome curves upward. The superior surface of the dome forms the floor of the thoracic cavity and the inferior surface of the dome forms the roof of the abdominal cavity.

As a dome, the diaphragm has peripheral attachments to structures that make up the abdominal and chest walls. The muscle fibers from these attachments converge in a central tendon, which forms the crest of the dome. Its peripheral part consists of muscular fibers that take origin from the circumference of the inferior thoracic aperture and converge to be inserted into a central tendon.

The muscle fibers of the diaphragm emerge from many surrounding structures. Anteriorly, fibers emerge from behind the xiphoid process and the cartilages of the floating ribs (ribs 7–12). Laterally, fibers emerge from the sides of the ribs

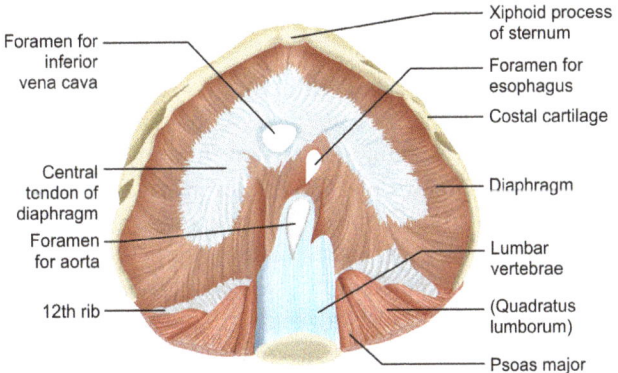

FIG. 9: Diaphragm.

themselves, including the two false ribs 11 and 12. Posteriorly, fibers emerge from the abdominal wall and lumbar vertebrae. There are two lumbocostal arches, medially and laterally.

Crura and central tendon: The left and right crura are tendinous in structure and blend with the anterior longitudinal ligament of the vertebral column.

The central tendon of the diaphragm is a thin but strong aponeurosis situated near the center of the vault formed by the muscle, but somewhat closer to the front than to the back of the thorax, so that the posterior muscular fibers are the longer. Once the diaphragm has been outlined, you can appreciate that the pleural gutter is deep posteriorly. Fluid, thus, tends to accumulate posteriorly.

Mediastinum (Fig. 10)

Mediastinum is the space between the lungs from inlet to outlet of thorax. Superiorly, by suprasternal notch. Anteriorly, it is in between parasternal lines. Posteriorly, by vertebral line. Inferiorly, it extends to xiphisternum. Mediastinum is narrow posteriorly and widens anteriorly. Since the inlet of thorax is slanted, only posterior mediastinum extends to neck.

Sternal angle separates superior from inferior mediastinum. The inferior mediastinum is divided into anterior, middle, and posterior compartments. The space in front of the heart is anterior mediastinum and behind is posterior mediastinum. Heart itself defines the middle mediastinum. The posterior mediastinum is divided into two, i.e., paravertebral and prevertebral space. Superior mediastinum extends into the neck and is called cervicomediastinal space.

It is important to know the structures in each compartment. It is important to differentiate the masses in the mediastinum in relation to the structures there.

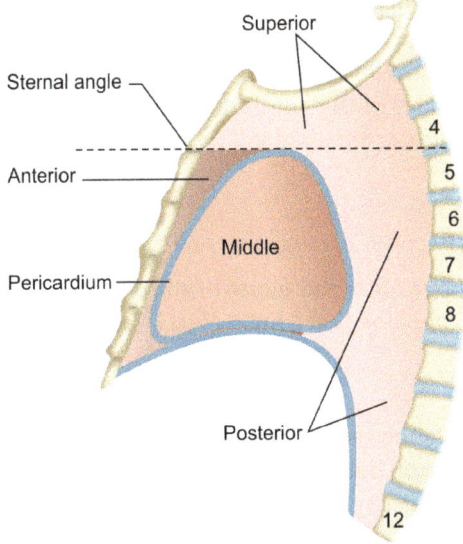

FIG. 10: Mediastinum.

Pleura and Pleural Sacs

Parietal and visceral pleura covers the surface of the lung. Parietal pleura lines inner surface of rib cage and outer portion of each hemidiaphragm is supplied by intercostal nerves and this is one reason for localized chest pain.

The pleura in the central region of each hemidiaphragm is innervated by fibers that travel with the phrenic nerve (C3–C4). So, in infection involving this area, the pain extends to ipsilateral neck or shoulder even to the abdomen presenting as acute abdomen. Parietal pleura has innervations and is pain sensitive but not the visceral pleura.

The pleural sac extends to 8th, 10th, and 12th rib in the midclavicular line, the midaxillary line, and scapular line, respectively at the lower level. There is a difference in the pleural reflection on the left side because the lung and the pleura from midsternal line lie at a higher level, i.e., at the lower border of the 4th costal cartilage. The superficial cardiac dullness is obtained in this area because the heart is uncovered.

Hilum

Hilum lies opposite to the spines of 4th, 5th, and 6th thoracic vertebrae. Left hilum is at a higher level.

Costal Angle

Costal angle (subcostal angle) is formed by the 10th rib with costal cartilage on both sides and xiphisternum in the middle. The normal angle is not >90° but more acute in males. Both the sides are symmetrical. Volume changes in each hemithorax will alter this relationship. Hyperinflated lungs will increase the costal angle. In alar chest, anterior–posterior distance is reduced. Diaphragmatic paralysis also alters the symmetry of costal angle.

Spinous Process

The most prominent spinous process is of 7th cervical vertebra. You can count down the thoracic vertebra and the ribs using this landmark.

To conclude, this chapter will throw light on the essentials of anatomy of thorax which will help in locating anatomical lesions with precession.

CHAPTER 2

Symptomatology

CARDINAL RULE TO HISTORY TAKING

The cardinal rule while presenting the history is "to avoid medical terms (one has to use the patients' words)."

The diseases of respiratory system may affect airways, lung, parenchyma, pleura, and the mediastinum.

Final diagnosis in respiratory medicine always has three parts (systemic disease to be excluded) that are as follows:
1. *Anatomical*: For example, right upper lobe, left lower lobe, pleura, etc.
2. *Pathological*: For example, fibrosis, bronchiectasis, cavity, effusion, pneumothorax, consolidation, etc.
3. *Etiological*: For example, tuberculosis, bacterial or viral pneumonias, etc.

When diagnosis is made, it should have the above three parts and if the patient is having any associated systemic illness such as hypertension, diabetes mellitus it has to be mentioned to make it a complete final diagnosis.

For example, right upper lobe bronchiectasis, post-tubercular with diabetes mellitus.

Common Symptoms

Common Respiratory Symptoms

- Cough—dry or wet (expectoration)
- Hemoptysis
- Breathlessness (dyspnea)
- Chest pain
- Hoarseness of voice
- Wheezing
- Stridor
- Sleep disturbances
- Dysphagia
- Sneezing, rhinitis
- Headache
- Allergy to certain food, flowers, dust, etc.

Constitutional Symptoms

- Fever
- Loss of weight
- Loss of appetite
- When the patient walks in, observe the patient (breathlessness, gait, facial expression, etc.). Ask the patient to be seated or make the patient lie down, if he is very sick.

Before the patient gives his/her complaints, note the following.

Proper History Taking

- *Name*:
- *Age*:
    - *Older age group*: Chronic bronchitis, lung cancer, and pulmonary tuberculosis (PTB).
    - *Younger age group*: Pulmonary tuberculosis, asthma.

- *Sex*:
  - Chronic obstructive pulmonary disease (COPD), carcinoma bronchus more in males.
  - Eventration of diaphragm, idiopathic pulmonary arterial hypertension (IPAH), and lymphangioleiomyomatosis (LAM) more in females.
- *Occupation*: Diseases such as silicosis, asbestosis, byssinosis, and hypersensitivity pneumonitis.
- *Race*: Asians are more prone to tuberculosis.
- *Recent history of travel*: Diseases in endemic areas (parasitic infections).
- *Residential address*: Near a factory, slum residents (environmental factors).

How to Proceed Further?

- *Presenting complaints (chief complaints)*: Note down the complaints in chronological order.
- *History of presenting illness*: Details (elaboration) of the above given symptoms in patient's words.
  - Past history
  - Family history
  - Personal history
  - Treatment history
  - Menstrual history in females

SYMPTOMS OF RESPIRATORY DISEASES

Common Respiratory Symptoms

Cough

Cough is the most common respiratory symptom. It is one of the most important defensive functions that protects the lower respiratory tract by preventing foreign material entering from outside and preventing stagnation of the secretions within the tract (pooling of secretions can lead to secondary infections and worsening of existing condition like bronchiectasis). Coughing is a response to any irritating stimuli from the level of pharynx down. By coughing, the irritants can be forcefully expelled. Coughing is a sudden expiration with closure of vocal cords. Cough reflex occurs as a result of the stimulation of the airway receptors.

Various types of cough have been described (common is dry or wet cough):
- Hacking dry cough—pharyngitis, smoker's cough
- Barking cough—croup, hysteria
- Brassy or metallic cough—mediastinal tumors, aortic aneurysm
- Paroxysmal cough
- Bovine cough—affliction of vocal cord.

Any cough lasting >2 weeks should be investigated. Worsening of cough in chronic bronchitis may be due to underlying lung malignancy. Sometimes, a bout of cough may produce sudden and transient loss of consciousness (cough syncope). Common causes and characteristics of cough are discussed in **Table 1**.

Cough can be dry or productive (with sputum production).

Dry Cough

No sputum production and the cough are irritating to the patient. Some of the conditions are mentioned above such as exposure to dust, postnasal drip, chronic pharyngitis, chronic laryngitis, foreign body, inhalation of irritant gases, smoker's cough, chronic sinusitis, foreign body, or wax in auditory meatus. Pressure on the airways as in aortic aneurysm, dilated left atrium, enlargement of mediastinal lymph nodes, retrosternal thyroid, and druginduced cough may be the other causes. In hysterical cough, there is no sputum production

TABLE 1: Common causes and characteristics of cough.

Common causes	Nature/character
Postnasal drip, usually irritate pharynx [now called as upper airway cough syndrome (UACS)]	Usually persistent
Laryngitis, whooping cough, croup, and tumor	Harsh, barking, painful, persistent associated with laryngeal tumor
Tracheitis	Painful
Bronchitis (acute and chronic)	Dry or productive, scanty, or more in the morning
Asthma	Dry or productive, more at night or after exposure to cold air or allergens. It can be more at night and early morning (diurnal variation) and may worsen with seasonal variation
Pulmonary tuberculosis	Associated with fever, loss of weight
Carcinoma bronchus	Persistent, often with hemoptysis
Bronchiectasis	Purulent, large quantity, occasional hemoptysis, postural dependence, and foul smell
Lung abscess	Same as bronchiectasis
Pneumonia	Dry initially, later productive
Pulmonary edema	Often at night, may be productive with pink frothy sputum
Interstitial lung disease	Dry irritating and distressing
Drug-induced (ACE inhibitor/β-blocker)	Dry and temporal association with the drug intake can be elicited
GERD	Dry, usually associated with other components of GERD such as belching, bloating, etc.

(ACE: angiotensin-converting enzyme; GERD: gastroesophageal reflux disease)

and the patient's attention is diverted (like asking rapid fire questions), the cough ceases, and patient will be able to speak normally.

Cough with Expectoration
- *Quantity*: Normally 10–20 mL of mucous is produced daily as it is a protective mechanism. This will help in ciliary movement which will help in clearing the airways of unwanted elements. Excess production will stimulate the respiratory mucous membrane and it will be expectorated out. It is better to encourage the patient to use the sputum cup, so that the patient will not spit in the open. Usually, the quantity is assessed in cup measurement (standard cup is approximately 200 mL). While taking ward rounds or during case taking, it is worthwhile to have a look at the sputum cup (opened!) which will yield a lot of information.

    Large quantities are seen in lung abscess, bronchiectasis, etc. Three-layered sputum can be demonstrated in the above conditions. The patient is asked to expectorate out the sputum in a glass jar and after 24 hours we may be able to appreciate three layers of sputum—the top most layer will be mucoid, middle layer will be mucopurulent, and bottom layer will be purulent. In olden days, importance was given to this observation, now replaced by X-ray and CT scans. In adenocarcinoma in situ, the quantity may be 2–3 L/24 h called bronchorrhea (how distressing!). In early stages of PTB, pneumonia, and acute and chronic bronchitis, the sputum may be scanty.
- *Color and appearance*:

Layman's terms	Medical jargon
White	Mucoid
Yellowish white	Mucopurulent indicates infection. Antibiotics may be given
Yellowish	Purulent. Definite infection. Antibiotics should be given

Infections can precipitate exacerbation of asthma, cor pulmonale, worsening of chronic bronchitis, bronchiectasis, etc. Here, antibiotics are definitely indicated without any delay.

- *Green color*: It commonly indicates *Pseudomonas* infections. Sometimes, normal individuals expectorate greenish sputum in the morning. It is due to the breakdown of leukocytes in the night and subsequent release of verdoperoxidase enzyme which gives the greenish color to the sputum. Unlike *Pseudomonas* infection, no treatment is required.
- *Rusty color*: In pneumonia, especially streptococcal pneumonia, during the stage of red hepatization, sputum has rusty color because of the destruction of the red blood cells (RBCs).
- *Anchovy sauce*: Hepatopulmonary amebiasis.
- *Red currant jelly*: *Klebsiella pneumonia.*
- *Pink and frothy*: Pulmonary edema.
- *Black or gray*: Smokers, industrial and atmospheric pollution, coal miners disease (pneumoconiosis), and bacterial or fungal infections (nocardiosis, aspergillosis).
- *Hemoptysis*: Will be discussed later.

- *Consistency*:
  - Thick and difficult to expectorate (chronic bronchitis).
  - Thin and watery (asthma).
- *Effect on changing position (postural variation)*: Patients with suppurative lung diseases such as bronchiectasis, lung abscess, etc., will have increased cough and sputum production with change in postures. So, they tend to adopt a position least distressing to them. For example, a patient with leftsided lesion prefers to lie on the same side and if he is asked to turn to right side he will start coughing and

bring out sputum. Because of the gravity, the secretions come to the major airways where the cough receptors are situated and patient coughs out the sputum, thus preventing pooling of secretions and secondary infection. We would like the patient to lie on the opposite side of the lesion (here right side) to clear away the secretions and postural drainage with the help of a physiotherapist, so as to prevent secondary infection.
- Associated chest pain while coughing (discussed later).
- *Foul-smelling sputum*: It is due to anaerobic organisms (*Peptostreptococcus, Fusobacterium, Bacteroides*) which produce short-chain fatty acids—butyrate or butyric acid. Seasonal and diurnal variation should be inquired.

Hemoptysis

It refers to coughing out blood. It may be a large quantity (aspergilloma), bronchiectasis, or streaking of sputum (carcinoma bronchus initial stage).

To remember: *The bleeding may not be necessarily from the lower respiratory tract*. It may be from nose (epistaxis), gums (gingivitis) leading to irritation of larynx or pharynx as postnasal drip or upper airway cough syndrome (UACS).

Causes

Respiratory
- Pulmonary tuberculosis
- Carcinoma bronchus
- Bronchiectasis—especially bronchiectasis sicca (dry bronchiectasis) where the patient will not have recurrent respiratory infections, but occasional hemoptysis. The lesions in the upper lobes have no pooling of secretions because of gravity.
- Aspergilloma

- Foreign body
- Lung abscess
- Benign lung tumors
- Trauma
- Pulmonary infarction
- Catamenial hemoptysis (occurs during menstruation)

Cardiovascular
- Mitral stenosis
- Pulmonary edema (pink frothy sputum)

Others
- Blood dyscrasias

Hemoptysis—quantification

- *Massive hemoptysis*: 600 mL or more in 24 hours as one episode or at different bouts or continuous hemoptysis of >100 mL/h for 3 hours or any amount which causes hemodynamic instability.
- *Moderate hemoptysis*: 50–200 mL in 24 hours.
- *Minimal hemoptysis*: Streaking of sputum with blood (carcinoma bronchus is an example) or 50 mL or less in 24 hours.

Most important cause of death in hemoptysis is due to aspiration and asphyxia rather than exsanguination. The differences between hemoptysis and hematemesis are discussed below in **Table 2**.

This differentiation is not the rule of thumb. Overlap can occur but still it is a useful guide. A detailed history taking is useful in distinguishing the two. Hemoptysis should be taken seriously even if it is minimal and investigated.

Spurious Hemoptysis

From upper respiratory tract (epistaxis, gingivitis, etc.) producing postnasal drip (UACS).

TABLE 2: Differences between hemoptysis and hematemesis.

Hemoptysis	Hematemesis
Coughing out blood	Vomiting blood
Bright red	Coffee colored or dark brown
Frothy	Mixed with food particles
Small quantity (not essential)	Large quantity
With coexisting chronic respiratory disease	Gastrointestinal (GI) disease
Malena absent	Malena present
pH alkaline	pH acidic
Bronchoscopy	Upper GI endoscopy

Pseudohemoptysis

Due to pigment prodigiosin produced by gram-negative organism—*Serratia marcescens*.

Endemic Hemoptysis

Produced by *Paragonimus westermani* (lung fluke).

Breathlessness or Dyspnea

When presenting the history, breathlessness only can be used as it is the layman's term (not dyspnea). Inquire about any relation to seasonal or diurnal variation.

Definition: Dyspnea is the unpleasant awareness of one's own breathing. It can be physiological; the reason being on severe exertion anyone can have breathlessness, which is unpleasant, but when dyspnea is present in a situation where it is *not due to physical exertion*, then it can be considered pathological and needs evaluation, e.g., like breathlessness at rest or taking a few steps.

Various grading systems are available—modified Medical Research Council (mMRC) (commonly used) and the New York Heart Association (NYHA). For simplicity and understanding, the following classification is useful.

Grading of Dyspnea

Teaching mMRC grading to undergraduate students is and will be difficult if we follow this new system (as they will be confused while reading this book). The previous grading is good enough to assess the severity of dyspnea.

- *Grade I*: On unaccustomed exertion. For example, everyday a normal person climbs two flights of stairs but if asked to climb four flights he will become breathless. This is an *unaccustomed* exertion.
- *Grade II*: On accustomed exertion. For example, the same person after a few years may not be able to climb two flights at a stretch and he may have to rest in between.
- *Grade III*: Minimal exertion such as bathing, walking a few steps, buttoning the shirt, etc., may produce breathlessness.
- *Grade IV*: Dyspnea at rest.

Clinically useful Classification

- *Dyspnea of sudden onset*: Pneumothorax, exacerbation of asthma, pulmonary embolism, pulmonary edema, foreign body in major airways, and inhalation of noxious gases.
- *Subacute dyspnea (progressing over weeks or months)*: Congestive cardiac failure, anemia, obesity, pleural effusion, ascites, pregnancy, and interstitial lung disease (ILD).
- *Chronic dyspnea (progressing over months or years)*: Chronic bronchitis, emphysema, pneumoconiosis, and pulmonary fibrosis (common in India due to PTB).

- *Dyspnea on exertion*: Anemia, pregnancy, pulmonary thromboembolism, mitral stenosis, chronic bronchitis, asthma, pulmonary fibrosis (ILD and PTB sequelae), kyphoscoliosis, and obesity.
- *Dyspnea at rest*:
  - Acute mechanical or infective condition
  - Pneumothorax, pleural effusion, pulmonary infarction, and pneumonia
  - Paroxysmal dyspnea
  - Pulmonary edema, asthma
  - Psychogenic
  - Hyperventilatory syndrome
  - Metabolic
  - Acidosis of uremia or diabetes (Kussmaul breathing)
  - Cheyne–Stokes breathing (hyperpnea and apnea) (as in cerebrovascular accidents)
  - Biot's breathing
  - Ondine's curse
- *Orthopnea*: The patient is more comfortable in sitting up and may become breathless on lying flat. It usually occurs in cardiac failure due to increase in left atrial pressure. It can occur in exacerbation of asthma, COPD, and ILD also.
- *Paroxysmal nocturnal dyspnea*: As the term indicates breathlessness occurs at night (early morning), as it is classically seen in cardiac conditions such as pulmonary edema (previously known as cardiac asthma) and asthma.
- *Platypnea*: Shortness of breath in upright position—arteriovenous malformation in lung as occurs in chronic liver disease (hepatopulmonary syndrome) or hereditary condition—atrial myxoma.
- *Orthodeoxia*: Oxygen desaturation in upright position which is >3%.
- *Trepopnea*: Breathlessness while lying on the side—cardiac causes, unilateral massive pleural effusion.

Chest Pain

Pain in the anterior part of the chest is an important symptom in respiratory and cardiac disorders and to be taken seriously.

When the patient complaints of chest pain, a detailed history taking is important. It may be either due to conditions such as *cellulitis, mastitis, premenstrual pain, myalgia, herpes, intercostal neuralgia, rib fractures, costochondritis* (Tietze syndrome) or due to serious causes such as *angina, myocardial infarction, pleuritic pain, gastroesophageal reflux disease, rib erosions, mediastinitis*, etc.

As far as this book is concerned, emphasis is given to chest pain secondary to pulmonary disorders. For example, pleurisy, pneumothorax, acute pulmonary embolism, pneumonia, massive collapse of the lung, lung abscess, bronchiectasis, carcinoma bronchus, pneumomediastinum, mediastinal growth, etc.

Pleuritic pain is usually localized (not diffuse), sharp and stabbing, dull ache, or felt as a "catch", aggravated by coughing, sneezing, laughing, crying, and deep breathing usually felt at the end of inspiration caused by inflamed pleura. The innervation of pleura is discussed earlier.

Patients with pleuritic pain often prefer lying on the side of pain or support the affected area with the hand (autosplinting).

Recurrent pleuritic pain can occur in bronchiectasis during infection.

Hoarseness of Voice

Patient notices change in voice. Common causes are pharyngitis, laryngitis, tuberculous laryngitis, larynx carcinoma, recurrent laryngeal nerve palsy, and inhaled corticosteroids producing myopathy of adductor muscles of the vocal cord, Ortner's syndrome.

Wheezing

Some patients may complain of abnormal or whistling noises produced in the chest while breathing as in the case of asthmatics or patients with chronic bronchitis, vocal cord dysfunction.

Stridor

This is a serious condition where upper airway obstruction occurs. It results from partial obstruction and narrowing of larynx, trachea. It is usually inspiratory and may be audible without a stethoscope.

Sleep Disturbances

Inquire about the patient's sleep pattern, snoring history and history of apneas—usually elicited from the bed partner, history related to obstructive sleep apnea, excessive daytime sleepiness, daytime fatigue, unrefreshing sleep, etc.

Other Symptoms

- *Dysphagia*: Compression of esophagus secondary to enlarged mediastinal node compression due to various pathological conditions (cannot include as a respiratory symptom exclusively).
- History of sneezing and rhinitis (seasonal variation), allergy to food, pollen, etc.

Constitutional Symptoms

Fever

Normal temperature is 36.6–37.2°C when taken orally, rectal temperature is 0.5–0.6°C higher, but axillary temperature is 0.5°C less. Usually rise in temperature above 37.2°C in the morning and above 37.7°C in the evening is taken as pyrexia. All individuals have a circadian rhythm with evening temperature of 0.5–1°C more than in the morning. A slight rise in temperature during ovulation can occur.

Types of Fever

- *Continuous*: Temperature is present throughout the day but never touches the baseline in 24 hours and the fluctuation is not >1°C.
- *Remittent*: Temperature never touches the baseline in 24 hours and the fluctuation is >2°C.
- *Intermittent*: Temperature touches the baseline at least once in 24 hours.
  Note: Evening rise of temperature described in tuberculosis is because of the increased levels of cytokines [interleukin-1 (IL-1)].

Loss of Appetite

Patient may not be eating well now as used to be earlier and they may have disinclination to take the food.

Loss of Weight

Patient or the relatives have noticed the loss of weight. In India, two most common causes for loss of weight are PTB or carcinoma bronchus.

Significant Weight Loss

Different authors give different percentage such as:
- 5% in 30 days.
- 7.5% in 60 days.
- 10% in 180 days.

HISTORY TAKING

Past History

Previous history of any illness might give us a clue regarding the present disease.

In respiratory medicine: *The must to know* are past history of asthma, allergic disorders, diabetes mellitus, hypertension, PTB (contact history), epilepsy (aspiration pneumonia), childhood history of measles, and whooping cough.

Family History

History of ILD, COPD, asthma, allergy, diabetes mellitus, hypertension, epilepsy (all this can be inherited), and history of symptoms suggestive of PTB in other family members should be elicited.

Personal History

Sleep, bowel and bladder habits, smoking (smoking index is number of cigarettes smoked per day × number of years), alcohol use, substance abuse, dietary habits, and spouse and children (pedigree chart) (**Fig. 1**).

Consanguineous marriage (marriage between individuals who are closely related) - consanguinity may have high risk of birth defects and abnormalities. A risk of autosomal

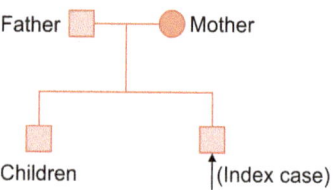

FIG. 1: Pedigree chart.

recessive disorders increases in offspring coming from consanguineous marriages due to the increased likelihood of receiving recessive genes from cognate parents. Inbreeding is associated with decreased cognitive abilities in children and still births and postnatal mortality.

Socioeconomic History

Judging socioeconomic status from dress, cleanliness is a questionable approach but may be useful in isolated cases which cannot be totally relied upon.

Treatment History

This may be elicited with the past history but patients with respiratory disorder volunteer even the specific names of the drugs like an asthmatic may say he is on salbutamol or aerosol therapy or a person who had tuberculosis may give the name of the drugs he had taken or say while taking the drugs urine was orange colored (rifampicin). History of surgery and anesthesia (aspiration pneumonia) should be taken. History of treatment for hypertension is important because angiotensin-converting enzyme (ACE) inhibitors produce dry cough.

Menstrual History

Must in all adult female patients, especially last menstrual period (LMP).

One of the most common causes of infertility in India is genitourinary tract tuberculosis. All types of menstrual irregularities can be encountered in genitourinary tuberculosis.

In endometriosis (ectopic endometrial tissue), as in thoracic endometriosis or endometriosis of the lung, the patient may have hemoptysis or pneumothorax during menstruation (rare).

Summarizing the History

After completing history taking, try to summarize the history (as some of the examiners will prefer to have only positive points from the history) to come to a provisional diagnosis.

MAKING PROVISIONAL DIAGNOSIS FROM HISTORY OBTAINED

Once the history taking is systematically done, we may be able to come to a differential diagnosis even before touching the patient (in nearly 80%).

Look at the examples given below.

CASE STUDY 1

A 45-year-old manual laborer with smoking habit, complaints of cough with scanty mucopurulent expectoration of 3 weeks duration with occasional hemoptysis for the last 7 days, streaky in nature. He has occasional fever and loss of weight. He was treated at a local hospital, but not relieved. He also has history of breathlessness for the last 5 years for which he takes occasional medication.

There is a past history of PTB, with no history of asthma, hypertension, diabetes, and epilepsy. There is no family history of any of the above conditions. There is a personal history of smoking (smoking index of 400), not an alcoholic, normal bowel and bladder habits, and consumes mixed diet. He is married and has two children. For the above symptoms, he was taking five injections from the local doctor with some syrup recently. He was getting treatment at the local hospital for breathlessness and recurrent respiratory infections for the last 5 years.

Differential Diagnosis from History
- Pulmonary tuberculosis
- Carcinoma bronchus
- Chronic obstructive pulmonary disease and increase in frequency of coughing or hemoptysis as an indicator for malignancy.
- Bronchiectasis (not the typical symptoms)

CASE STUDY 2

A 50-year-old male patient, a quarry worker was brought to the casualty with coughing out yellowish white sputum, hemoptysis and fever of 5 days duration. Blood was bright red in color and frothy, about 100 mL in 24 hours. He was apparently alright 5 days back. He had no associated complaints. He gave past history of taking antitubercular treatment 3 years back and had completed the full course. There is no past history of asthma, diabetes, hypertension, epilepsy, or aspiration. There is no family history of asthma, diabetes, hypertension, or epilepsy.

Personal History: Smoker, alcoholic, and bowel and bladder habits are normal. Consumes mixed diet.

Treatment history of tuberculosis (intermittent regimen), completed 6 months of treatment 3 years back.

Differential Diagnosis from History
- Reactivation of PTB
- Silicotuberculosis
- Bronchiectasis
- Carcinoma bronchus
- Pneumonia
- Lung abscess

CASE STUDY 3

A 38-year-old asthmatic lady was admitted with the complaints of left-sided chest pain, cough with yellowish sputum, fever, and increasing breathlessness in spite of her regular medications since 10 days. On further questioning, she had also complaints of loss of appetite and loss of weight. Her relatives also noticed change in her voice. She is asthmatic from childhood and on regular treatment with metered-dose inhalers. No history of diabetes, hypertension, epilepsy, and no history of taking antitubercular treatment.

Family history of asthma, diabetes, but no history of hypertension, epilepsy, or PTB.

Personal History: Normal bowel and bladder habits. She has normal appetite with fewer intakes now. She is married and has one child. Her spouse and child are healthy according to her.

She is using inhaled corticosteroids and long-acting β2 agonist for the last 2 years. Before that, she was on oral bronchodilators. Her menstrual cycle is irregular and with excessive bleeding.

Differential Diagnosis from History

- Acute severe asthma secondary to infection.
- Pneumothorax (left)
- Pulmonary tuberculosis. Long history of asthma, already on inhaled steroids, and probably would have taken oral corticosteroids knowingly or unknowingly with probable genital tuberculosis (irregular periods).
- Hoarseness of voice may be due to acute or chronic pharyngitis, laryngitis, and tubercular laryngitis or she was not instructed to wash the mouth and gargle after using inhaled corticosteroids. This may lead to myopathy of adductor muscles of vocal cord.
- Pneumonia
- Pleural effusion (left)
- To rule out diabetes mellitus (family history of diabetes and probably secondary to chronic steroid use).

CHAPTER 3

Examination of Respiratory System

INTRODUCTION

- Orientation to time, place, and person (this will give us an idea about patient's conscious level).
- Build and nourishment
- *Anthropometry*:
  - Height
  - Weight
  - Upper and lower segment ratio
  - Calculation of body mass index (BMI).

Warm your hands before touching the patient and inform the patient what you are going to do.

VITAL SIGNS

- *Temperature*: Normal temperature is 36.6–37.2°C. *Temperature was discussed in detail while dealing with symptomatology.*
- *Pulse*: Usually radial pulse is palpated. Normal is taken as 70 and 80 beats/min while resting (may vary with sex, age, and body build). Examiner has to check for—rate, rhythm, volume, character, force, condition of arterial

wall, radial-femoral delay, examining peripheral pulse, check for left and right radial pulse to know that they are equal (difference may be there in coarctation of the aorta, aortitis, and peripheral embolism).
- *Respiratory rate*: Assess the following—rate, rhythm, type, and use of accessory muscles. Normal—16–20 breaths/min while resting. The respiration pulse ratio is roughly calculated as 1:4.

  Inspiration is an active process whereas expiration is a passive process. The type of respiration in males is usually abdominothoracic and in females it is thoracoabdominal type and in disease conditions, the type may alter (refer page 54).
- *Blood pressure*: Normal systolic pressure is 120 mm Hg and normal diastolic pressure is 80 mm Hg at rest and variation can occur with age. The readings may vary with the time of the day, anxiety, temperature, etc.
- *Pulse oximetry* (now portable pulse oximeter is available)—to measure oxygen saturation (SpO_2).

GENERAL PHYSICAL EXAMINATION

Examine for pallor, icterus, cyanosis, lymphadenopathy, clubbing, pedal edema, jugular venous pulse (JVP), and any scars on the visible part of the body [this may give us a clue regarding pleural tap, implantable cardioverter defibrillator (ICD) insertion scars, thoracotomy scars, "branding scars", etc.].

Pallor

Pallor is very common and can be appreciated when palpebral conjunctiva is examined. It may be due to blood loss secondary to hookworm infestation, severe hemoptysis, hematemesis, and menorrhagia. There will be individual variation, so anemia can only diagnosed after getting the hemoglobin report. Pallor can be due to shock also—patient need not have anemia.

Suffused conjunctiva may be due to secondary polycythemia or superior vena cava obstruction.

Icterus

Bulbar conjunctiva is to be examined for yellowish discoloration—icterus, again the interpretation is subjective. So, serum bilirubin report will be confirmatory. The patient has to be examined in daylight and not artificial light. Muddy conjunctiva can mislead.

Cyanosis

Bluish discoloration of the skin and the mucous membrane due to an increase in the amount of reduced hemoglobin in the capillary bed in excess of 5 g/100 mL. It is of three types.

Central Cyanosis

Causes

- *Decreased arterial oxygen saturation*:
  - High altitude
  - Impaired pulmonary function [chronic obstructive pulmonary disease (COPD), asthma, diffuse pulmonary lung disease, and pneumonia].
  - Anatomic shunts—cyanotic congenital heart disease, pulmonary arteriovenous fistula, and intrapulmonary shunts.
  - Hemoglobin with low affinity for oxygen [hemoglobin Kansas (HbK)].

- *Hemoglobin abnormality*:
  - *Methemoglobinemia*:
    - Hereditary
    - *Acquired*: Drug-induced—nitrates and sulfonamide
  - Sulfhemoglobinemia
  - Carboxyhemoglobinemia (smokers)

Peripheral Cyanosis

Causes

- Reduced cardiac output.
- Cold exposure
- Redistribution of blood flow from extremities.
- Arterial and venous obstruction

Differential Cyanosis

Causes

- Patent ductus arteriosus (PDA) with pulmonary arterial hypertension with right-to-left shunt—cyanosis is seen in lower limbs.
- Patent ductus arteriosus with pulmonary arterial hypertension with right-to-left shunt and transposition of the great vessels—cyanosis is seen in upper limbs.

Differentiating Features between Central and Peripheral Cyanosis

Central Cyanosis

Also seen in lips; whole body may be bluish—look at the nails and under the tongue, this is due to right-to-left shunt or due to diseases of lung. Extremities are warm and may be associated with clubbing or polycythemia. Oxygen inhalation may show marginal improvement, if it is an isolated pulmonary cause only and partial pressure of arterial oxygen (PaO_2) is usually low.

Peripheral Cyanosis

Cold, clammy extremities, with bluish discoloration of nail bed, nose tip, and earlobe. It occurs due to peripheral stasis and also seen in low cardiac output state. Bluish discoloration disappears on warming. No change with oxygen inhalation and PaO_2 is normal.

Lymphadenopathy

It can be generalized or localized. The sites generally looked for the presence of node enlargement are supraclavicular, scalene, axillary, submental, submaxillary, submandibular, preauricular, posterior auricular, and inguinal.

When examining for supraclavicular node, the subject is to be seated upright and examined from behind.

For scalene node, place the index finger between clavicle and sternocleidomastoid muscle and press down toward the first rib with the head slightly tilted to same side. The node is usually involved secondary to malignancy.

Tuberculous Lymphadenopathy

Usually affects cervical lymph node, but may affect axillary, inguinal, etc. They may be initially firm and freely mobile and later become soft, immobile, and matted together and adherent to skin and adjacent structures, sometimes with sinus formation and cold abscess.

Malignancy of Lung

Stony hard, usually supraclavicular and scalene node. If axillary node enlargement is present, suspect chest wall involvement by malignancy.

Virchow's Node

Troisier's sign—usually seen in the left supraclavicular fossa. It occurs in carcinoma of the lungs, stomach, kidney, or testis.

Acquired Immunodeficiency Syndrome

Persistent generalized lymphadenopathy with symmetrical, mobile, and nontender. Nodes usually affected are cervical, supraclavicular, submandibular, and axillary nodes.

Lymphomas

Rubbery, nontender lymph nodes in the neck.

Clubbing

It refers to the enlargement of the terminal phalanges of the digits due to increased subungual soft tissue.

Many theories have been attributed to clubbing such as humoral, neurogenic, hypoxia, decreased ferritin, and platelet-derived growth factor.

Lovibond's Angle

The angle between the nail and nail bed is normally 160° but in clubbing as illustrated in **Figure 1** it will increase.
- *Grade I*: Increased glossiness of skin over the nail bed.
- *Grade II*: Obliteration of the angle between the nail and nail bed and fluctuation will be present.

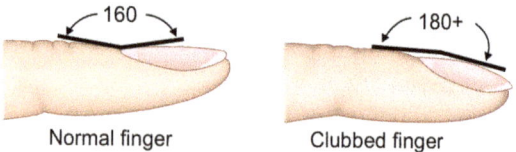

FIG. 1: Lovibond's angle.

- *Grade III*: Parrot beak appearance.
- *Grade IV*: Drumstick appearance and hypertrophic pulmonary periosteoarthropathy (HPPOA) [previously known as hypertrophic pulmonary osteoarthropathy (HPOA)].

Schamroth's Sign

It refers to sign when the dorsal part of the distal phalanges of fingers of both the hands is approximated to each other (**Fig. 2**). In normal subject, a diamond-shaped window is formed but in clubbing, it will be absent.

Interphalangeal Depth and Distal Phalangeal Depth

It is also a useful sign to diagnose clubbing. This can be appreciated by viewing from the side and ask the patient to spread the fingers. In normal individual, the interphalangeal depth (IPD) will be more than the distal phalangeal depth (DPD) (**Fig. 3A**), but in clubbing DPD will be more because of the increased curvature (**Fig. 3B**).

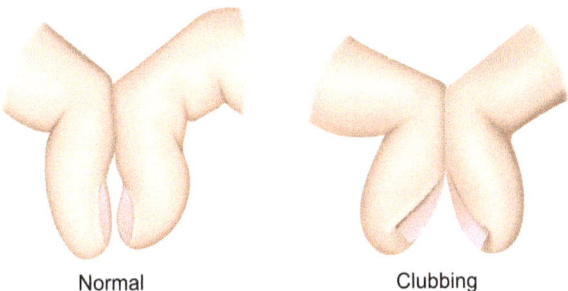

FIG. 2: Schamroth's sign.

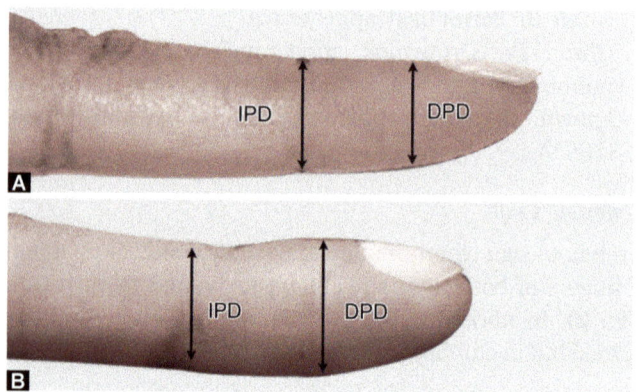

FIGS. 3A AND B: Interphalangeal depth (IPD) and distal phalangeal depth (DPD). (A) In normal individual; and (B) In case of clubbing.

Profile Sign

Ask the patient to spread the fingers and the examiner has to view from the side (the profile view).

Causes of Clubbing

Respiratory System

- Suppurative lung diseases (lung abscess, empyema, and bronchiectasis)
- Diffuse parenchymal lung disease
- Bronchogenic carcinoma
- Metastatic lung cancer
- Mesothelioma
- Sarcoidosis
- Pulmonary arteriovenous malformation

Cardiovascular System

- Congenital cyanotic heart disease
- Atrial myxoma

- Bacterial endocarditis
- Eisenmenger's syndrome

Gastrointestinal System
- Primary biliary cirrhosis
- Crohn's disease
- Ulcerative colitis
- Gastrointestinal malignancy

Other Causes
- Acromegaly
- Thyrotoxicosis
- Syphilis
  Familial clubbing is not common.

Other Less Common Conditions
- *Unidigital clubbing*: Gout, sarcoidosis, and local injury.
- *Unilateral clubbing*: Pancoast tumor, brachial arteriovenous fistula, aneurysmal dilatation of aorta, and subclavian or innominate arteries.
- *Differential clubbing*: Seen with PDA with reverse shunt—with cyanosis and clubbing of toes and left hand.
- *Pseudoclubbing*: Hyperparathyroidism, occupational (vinyl chloride workers), leprosy, and leukemia.

Pedal Edema

Usually, pitting type as seen in congestive cardiac failure, hypoproteinemia, and chronic renal failure. Demonstrated by pressing the finger a little above the middle malleolus/an inch or two above for few seconds and releasing the finger will show pitting. The upper extent of pedal edema can also be assessed by gradually assessing the shin of tibia below upward, but myxedema and chronic lymphedema due to filariasis are nonpitting.

Jugular Venous Pulse

Engorgement and visible pulsation of neck veins are abnormal above the level of manubrium sterni in sitting up or 45° from horizontal, i.e., semi-propped up position. External jugular vein is superficial but internal jugular vein is deep-seated and in direct line with the right atrium, usually the pulsation is seen beneath the sternocleidomastoid muscle.

Patient should be reclined at 45° in good daylight. Patient has to rest his head on a pillow to relax neck muscles and rotate the head slightly away from the side under observation. Look across the neck and identify internal jugular pulsation. Estimate the vertical height in centimeters between the top of jugular pulsation and sternal angle. Mean right atrial pressure is normally >7 mm Hg.

Since the sternal angle is approximately 5 cm above right atrium, the normal JVP should not extend >4 cm above the sternal angle.

Abdominojugular reflux—is the distension of the neck veins precipitated by the maneuver of firm pressure over the liver. It is seen in tricuspid regurgitation, heart failure due to other nonvalvular causes, and other conditions including constrictive pericarditis, cardiac tamponade, and inferior vena cava obstruction.

Causes of Increased Jugular Venous Pulse

- Cor pulmonale
- Hyperkinetic circulatory states—fever, pregnancy, and hyperthyroidism.
- Raised intrathoracic or intra-abdominal pressure—obesity, pregnancy, ascites, and pleural effusion.
- Obstructive lesions of vessel—superior vena cava obstruction.

EXAMINATION OF RESPIRATORY SYSTEM

Upper Respiratory Tract

Examination should be done in daylight or with aid of torch. It is preferable to do all components of respiratory examination on a bare chest.

Oral cavity: Look for:
- Lips—cyanosis, pallor, pursed lip breathing, angioedema, cheilitis, and herpes labialis.
- Teeth—caries, erosion, and anomalies.
- Gingivitis—bleeding gums.
- Buccal mucosa—leukoplakia, candidiasis, and Koplik's spots.
- Tongue—pallor, cyanosis, fiery red tongue, stomatitis, leukoplakia, coated tongue, and thrush.
- Palate—cleft palate, high-arched palate, ulcers, and tumors.
- Tonsils—swelling and abscess.
- Posterior pharyngeal wall—congestion.
- Uvula—any deviation of uvula.

Nose: Saddle nose, use of alae nasi, nasal discharge, epistaxis, deviated nasal septum, polyps, and turbinate hypertrophy.

Ears: Discharge, discoloration, and wax.

Lower Respiratory Tract

Inspection

- *Size, shape, and type of chest*: The normal adult chest is more or less bilaterally symmetrical, ellipsoidal, or conical in shape and elliptical in cross-section. The transverse diameter is greater than anteroposterior diameter

(7:5 ratio) and the vertical diameter exceeding both anteroposterior and lateral diameters with subcostal angle of 90° (acute in males) (**Fig. 4**).

- *Chest wall symmetry*:
  Symmetrical types of abnormal chest:
  - Flat chest—rickets
  - Alar chest
  - Pectus excavatum—cobbler's chest and Marfan syndrome (**Fig. 5**).
  - Pectus carinatum (pigeon chest)—rickets (**Fig. 6**).
  - Barrel chest—emphysema (**Fig. 7**).

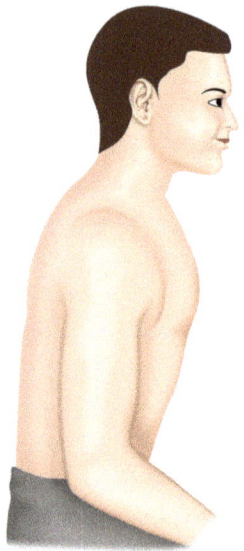

FIG. 4: Normal.

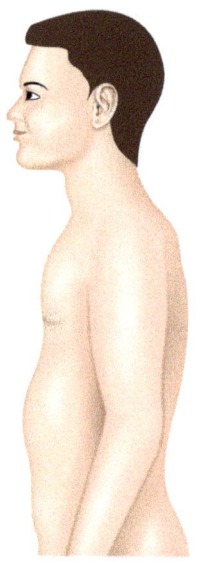

FIG. 5: Pectus excavatum.

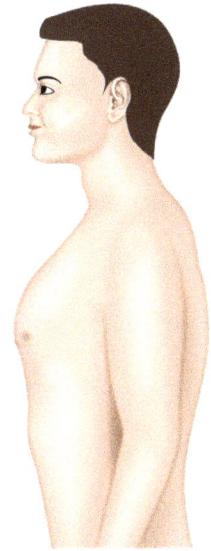

FIG. 6: Pectus carinatum.

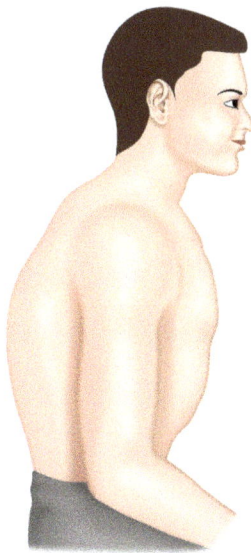

FIG. 7: Barrel shaped.

Asymmetrical types of abnormal chest:
- Unilateral flattening, retraction, drooping of shoulder (**Fig. 8**), hollowing of supraclavicular and infraclavicular fossae, crowding of ribs or spaces—collapse of lung, fibrosis, and wasting of muscles.
- Unilateral bulging—pneumothorax, pleural effusion, and any intrathoracic or extrathoracic swelling.
- Spinal abnormalities—kyphosis, scoliosis, and kyphoscoliosis (**Figs. 9** and **10**).

All these can later on lead to respiratory or cardiovascular complications.

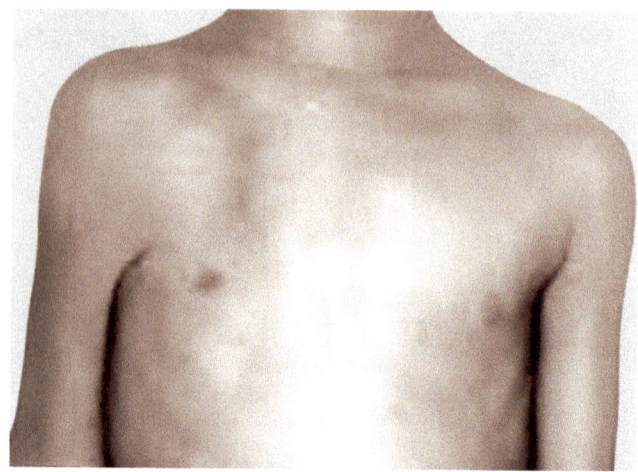

FIG. 8: Drooping of shoulder.

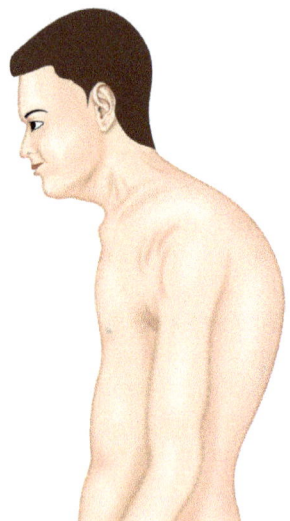

FIG. 9: Kyphosis.

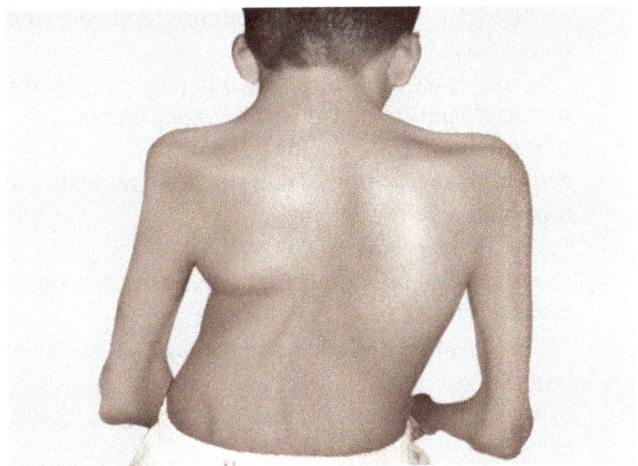

FIG. 10: Scoliosis.

Look for the presence of: Any engorged vessels, pulsations; intercostal retractions, movement of subcostal angle, use of accessory muscles, and types of breathing.

Inspect the position of:
- Trachea
- Apex beat
  Look for diaphragmatic movement.
- *Respiratory movements*: Normal respiratory rate is 16–20 breaths/min in adults.

  Types of breathing:
  - Thoracoabdominal in females.
  - Abdominothoracic in males.

  Abnormalities in respiration:
  - *Increased rate*: Tachypnea in exacerbations of asthma, COPD, and tension pneumothorax.

- - *Decreased rate*: Narcotic poisoning, diabetic coma, and uremia.
  - *Cheyne–Stokes breathing*: Narcotic poisoning, carbon monoxide poisoning, and central sleep apnea.
  - *Biot's breathing*: Meningitis
  - *Kussmaul breathing*: Diabetic ketoacidosis and metabolic acidosis.
  - *Pursed lip breathing*: COPD
  - *Rapid shallow breathing*: Restrictive lung disease and pleuritic chest pain.
  - *Ataxic breathing*: Brainstem damage at medullary level.
  - *Apneustic breathing*: Brainstem damage at pontine level.
  - *Stridor*: Laryngeal spasm, vocal cord paralysis, and malignant growth in trachea.
  - *Sleep disordered breathing*: Apnea and hypopnea
- *Thoracic movements*:
  - *Diminished bilaterally*: Emphysema, ankylosing spondylitis, and myasthenia gravis.
  - *Diminished unilaterally*: Lung collapse, pleural effusion, pneumothorax, and fibrosis.
  - *Intercostal indrawing*: Collapse of lung, fibrosis, and can be seen in exacerbations of asthma, COPD also.
  - *Hoover's sign*: Paradoxical movement of costal margin during inspiration seen in emphysema.
- *Position of apical impulse*: It is half an inch medial to midclavicular line on the left side at the level of 5th intercostal space.
- *Sternocleidomastoid sign (Trail's sign)*:
  - *Trail's sign (**Fig. 11**)*: It refers to the undue prominence of the clavicular head of sternocleidomastoid on the side to which trachea is shifted. The pretracheal fascia

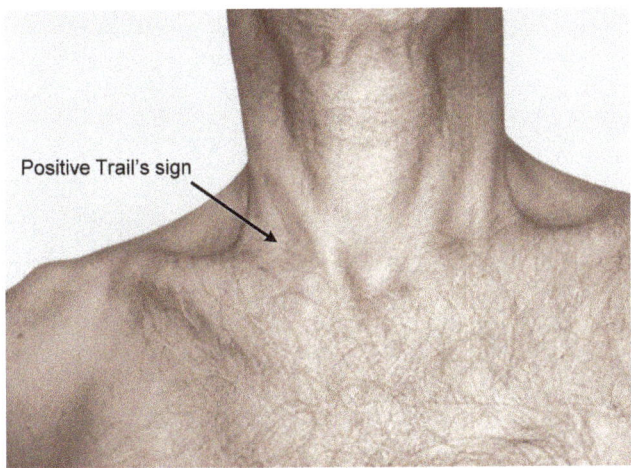

FIG. 11: Sternocleidomastoid sign (Trail's sign).

encloses the clavicular head of sternocleidomastoid on both sides. The clavicular head becomes prominent due to relaxation of pretracheal fascia where the trachea is shifted. Trachea is usually centrally placed, but it may deviate to left or right in fibrosis, collapse pneumothorax, pleural effusion fibrothorax, and large mass. It indicates the shift of the upper mediastinum.
- Distended chest veins, pulsating vessels, sinus, and scars.

Palpation

Palpate abnormal pulsation on the chest wall, abnormal swellings—lipoma, sebaceous cyst, and tumors involving chest wall.

Confirm inspection findings such as:
- *Position of trachea*: If the patient is sitting, stand in front of the patient and fix your ring and index finger on the

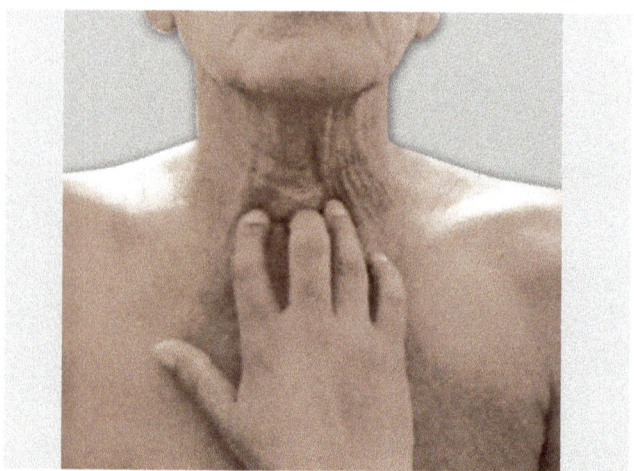

FIG. 12: Palpation of trachea.

prominence of the medial ends of both clavicles and gently run the middle finger down the trachea. If the trachea is central, the finger will come down in a straight line, but any deviation of trachea to left or right, the finger will slide in the direction where trachea is deviated (**Fig. 12**).

Another method is to push gently your finger between the trachea and medial end of sternocleidomastoid muscle and resistance is felt where the trachea is shifted.

- *Apical impulse*: The impulse is usually felt half an inch (1.25 cm) medial to the midclavicular line in the 5th intercostal space over the left side. Keep the palm of the hand where apical pulsation is seen on inspection with a little tilt of the patient to usually left side and then locate with the finger for the exact location.

  It indicates the shift of the lower mediastinum. Always remember dextrocardia where the apex beat is visualized on the right side.

Palpate for widening or narrowing of intercostal space and look for tenderness which may indicate empyema thoracis, subphrenic abscess, fracture, and Tietze syndrome.

- *Respiratory movements*: On inspection, respiratory movement is already observed preferably from the foot end and the finding may be subjective if there is not much difference in the movement of left and right hemithorax.

So, to confirm, palpation is required and follows these three steps:

1. *For apical region*: While the patient is seated with the head bent downward, the examiner has to stand behind the patient with both the hands placed over the apical region with thumbs to be kept besides the other fingers; comparison of the upward movement of the hands on both sides to be observed and in case of fibrosis, collapse—the movement may be reduced on the affected side (**Fig. 13A**).

   In lying down position, the hands are to be placed over the clavicles and note the movement of the hand while the patient takes deep inspiration. Also, the difference in movement can be appreciated by keeping the hands on either side of the neck and assess which hand moves higher.

2. *For the middle and lower regions (interscapular and infrascapular areas)*: The patient to be seated with hands crossed over the chest wall and slightly bending forward. The two hands of the examiner who is standing behind are placed symmetrically on either side of the patient's chest and this will help to grip the two sides with the palms and thumbs are opposed to meet in the midline. So, while the patient is breathing, the thumbs move away from midline normally, but in case of less movement of the thumb on one side, restriction of movement on the affected side

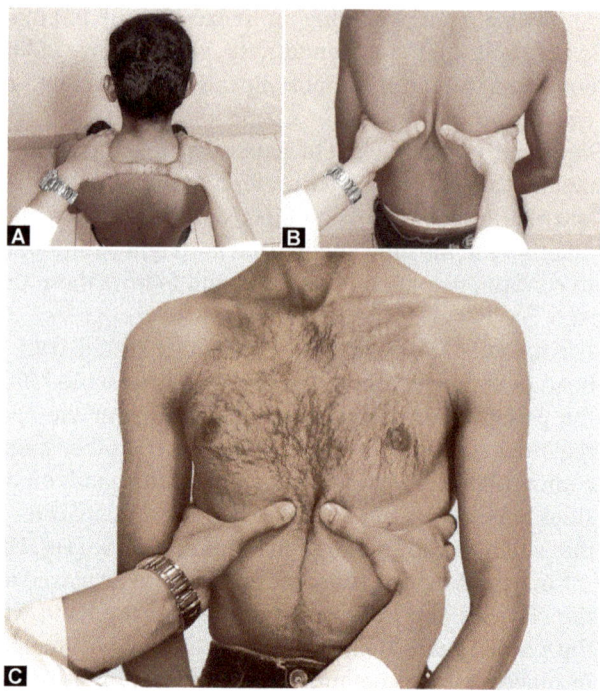

FIGS. 13A TO C: Chest wall expansion by palpation. (A) Apical; (B) Posterior; and (C) Anterior.

is suspected. Patient should be asked to inspire deeply (**Fig. 13B**).

3. *Anterior examination*: Keep the palm of both the hands in the 4th or 5th intercostal space and thumbs are opposed to meet in the midline. Ask the patient to take deep inspiration, the thumbs move away from midline normally, but in case of less movement of the thumb on one side, restriction of movement on the affected side is suspected (**Fig. 13C**).

In males, usually abdominothoracic type of respiratory movement is seen and in females, thoracoabdominal type of respiratory movement is seen. To appreciate this, when the patient is breathing, keep one hand over the chest and other hand over the abdomen. In males, the hand kept over the abdomen will move first and in females, the hand kept over the chest will move first.

- *Measurement of chest expansion*: The normal circumferences of the chest are taken first with a tape and then the patient is asked to take a deep inspiration and the difference is noted (**Fig. 14**).

Normal expansion is 5–8 cm, but in certain conditions it will be less.

Conditions of decreased expansion may be due to pleural effusion, pneumothorax, collapse, fibrosis, etc.

Spinoscapular distance is measured from the angle of scapula to the spine and distance is reduced considerably in fibrothorax.

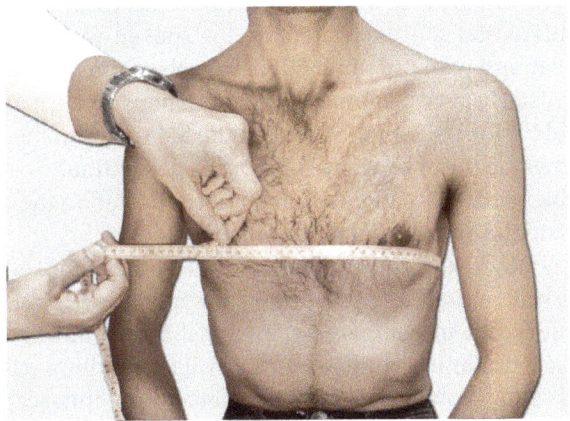

FIG. 14: Measurement of chest expansion.

- Diaphragmatic movement.
- *Tracheal descent with inspiration (tracheal tug)*: Cricosternal distance is a good indicator of tracheal descent. The normal cricosternal distance is three fingers (4–5 cm). Distance less than three fingers during inspiration indicate hyperinflation of lung.
- *Vocal fremitus*: Usually in a normal subject, low-frequency sound is transmitted to chest wall after it gets filtered by alveoli. In certain diseases, it may alter.

When a person produces a sound, there is vibration of chest wall. Larynx vibrates during phonation. The vibrating element is the vocal cords. This vibration is modified by the mouth, nose, nasal sinus, pharynx, and chest cavity (resonators). Thus, sound produced in larynx is transmitted to chest wall as vibration and the examiner can appreciate the vibrations by using the ulnar border of the palm kept on the chest wall to appreciate tactile vocal fremitus.

The patient is asked to say some number in their language (usually one..one..one) which should be distinct and patient is asked to repeat it when the examiner keeps the hand in the intercostal spaces, bilaterally. The spoken words should be clear and with the same intensity – place the hand in the intercostals spaces comparing the vibrations in each space, e.g., place the palm of the hand on the 3rd space on the right and then on the 3rd space left for better perception.

The words the patient uttered are conducted to the chest wall and the examiner feels the vibration.

Examiner keeps the ulnar border of the hand on the chest wall and tell the patient to say some number and the examiner has to compare symmetrical areas starting from supraclavicular to mammary areas, axillary and infra-axillary areas, and suprascapular, interscapular, and infrascapular areas (**Figs. 15** and **16** for points of reference for percussion).

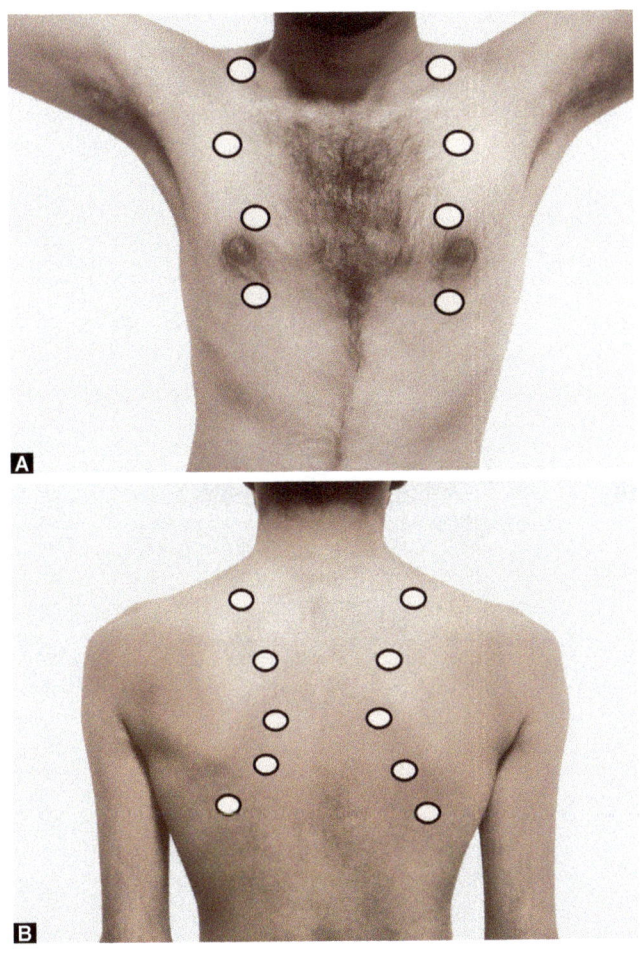

FIGS. 15A TO D: *(Continued)*

(Continued)

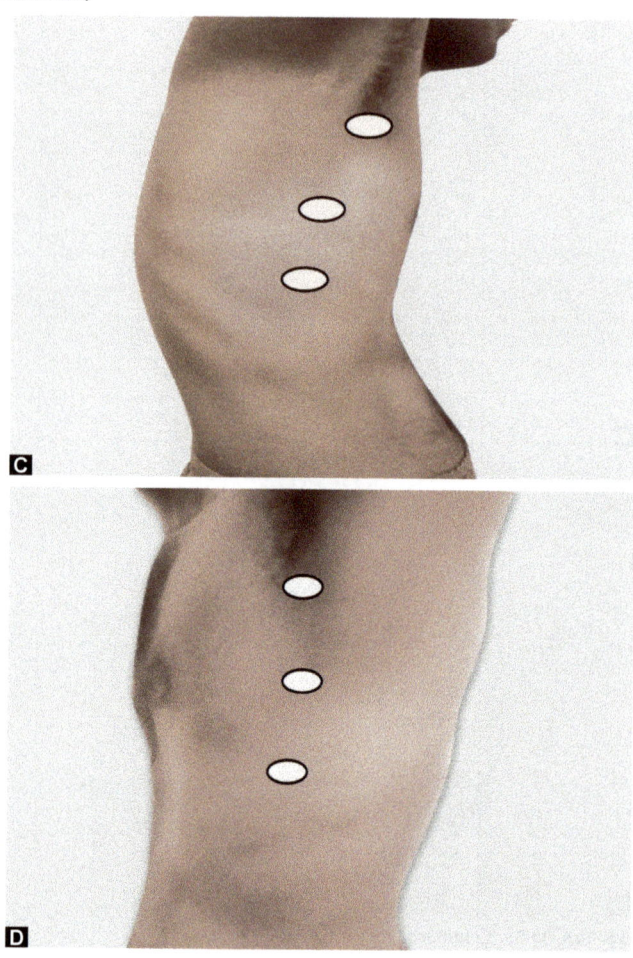

FIGS. 15A TO D: Vocal fremitus—topographical areas. (A) Anterior chest wall; (B) Posterior chest wall; (C) Right lateral; and (D) Left lateral.

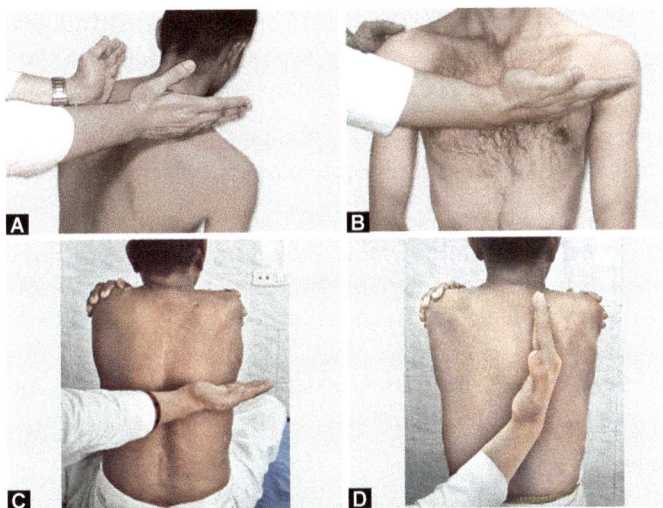

FIGS. 16A TO D: Vocal fremitus examination.

Tactile vocal fremitus is increased in consolidation, fibrosis and reduced in pleural effusion, pneumothorax, and lung collapse. Friction fremitus—palpable rub in pleurisy and palpable crepitus as in subcutaneous emphysema.

Percussion

By percussing the chest, we will hear the sound produced which is expressed as:
- Normal resonance
- Hyperresonant
- Impaired resonance or dull note
- Stony dull note
- Tympanitic note
- Subtympanitic

Percussion is also useful in marking the borders of lung, so as to make out whether there is hyperinflation (emphysema) or shrinkage of lung (collapse or fibrosis).

Two points to remember are: (1) Auditory perception of sound elicited; and (2) Tactile perception of the sense of resistance felt.

Position of patient: Preferably sitting down and not supine because the bed may dampen the sound. But if the patient is in supine position, percussion is carried out in both right and left lateral position.

Start percussion from supraclavicular area in front and from suprascapular area behind.

Anterior Percussion
- Hands on patient's hip (**Fig. 17**).

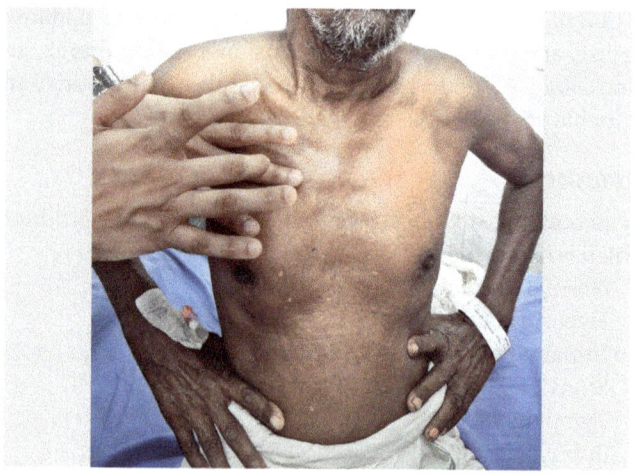

FIG. 17: Anterior percussion.

Posterior Percussion

- For suprascapular percussion, patient's hands are crossed on the thighs and patient is slightly stooping forward but relaxed.
- For the interscapular and infrascapular areas, patient is asked to keep the hands crossed on the shoulders (**Fig. 18**).

Lateral Percussion

- Hands over the head.

Cardinal Rules of Percussion

- Percussion should be done from resonant to dull areas.
- The examiner should be close to the patient and carefully listen to percussion note.
- Plexor finger is the tip of right middle finger which is used to strike the middle phalanx of pleximeter finger kept on

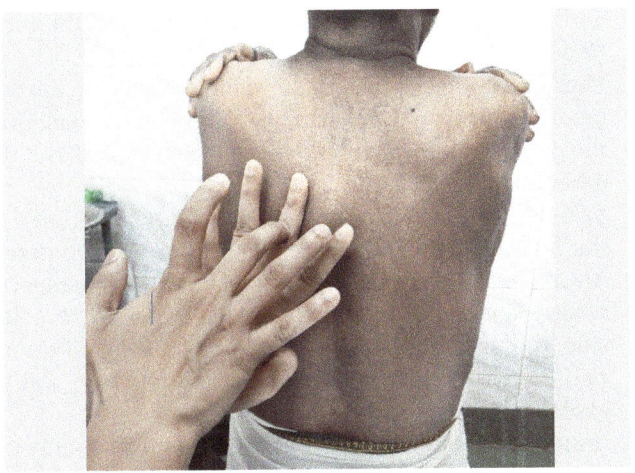

FIG. 18: Posterior percussion.

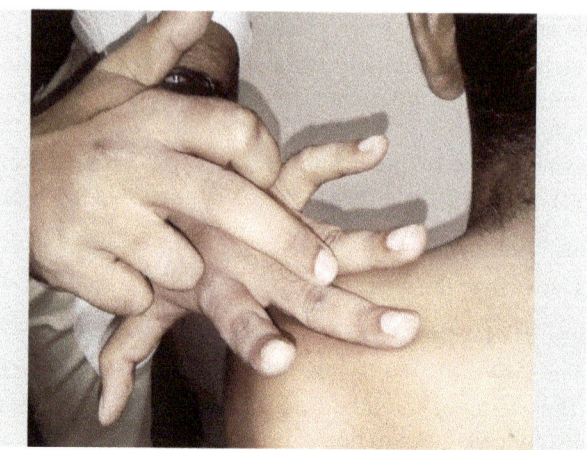

FIG. 19: Plexor finger to strike the middle phalanx of pleximeter finger.

the chest wall. Plexor finger acts like a hammer to strike and it should strike the pleximeter finger at right angle (**Fig. 19**).
- Pleximeter finger—that is the middle finger of the left hand kept firm on the chest wall to avoid air pockets. Only the pleximeter finger should touch the chest wall, not the other fingers.
- Symmetrical areas should be percussed anteriorly in the left and right interspaces and notes are compared. Always keep the pleximeter finger in the interspaces while percussing anteriorly and laterally. On the left side, presence of heart, stomach, and spleen and on the right liver may vary the percussion note (which will be explained later).
- Important to remember is that while percussing, only the wrist of the right hand should move and not the elbow.

- Each stroke must be sudden and withdraw the plexor immediately to avoid dampening of the note.
- Each stroke should produce a clear audible note and it may be difficult to demonstrate in obese patients.
- While percussing to demarcate the area of liver or heart, the long axis of the pleximeter finger must be kept parallel to the expected border of the organ.

Direct Percussion

The pleximeter finger is not used, but uses the plexor to percuss.

Clavicular Percussion

It may be useful in detecting lesions in the upper lobe. It is percussed on the medial third of clavicle. While percussing, the skin over the clavicle should be stretched by the index and middle finger of the other hand.

Sternal Percussion

Usually, dull note is produced by the presence of heart. But in case, the heart is shifted to left or right due to fibrothorax with hyperinflation or collapse, sternal percussion will be resonant.

Areas to be Percussed
- Supraclavicular
- Infraclavicular
- Mammary
- Axillary
- Infra-axillary
- Suprascapular
- Interscapular
- Infrascapular

Kronig's isthmus: It is a band area of resonance over each shoulder connecting zones of lung resonance over anterior and posterior aspects of both the sides of the chest apex. It is bounded anteriorly by clavicle, posteriorly by trapezius muscle, laterally by acromion process of scapula, and medially by neck structures. It is 5–7 cm in width and is resonant. But in the presence of a tumor or any other abnormality in the apex of upper lobe, it may become dull or impaired note can be elicited.

Types of Percussion Note

- *Normal resonant note*:
  - The normal percussion note in the chest is resonant due to vibration of air in the underlying lung tissue with millions of alveoli and of low pitch and clear in character (like tapping an empty metal box).
  - Resonant note is better heard in the front of chest wall (not in females) than the back. In the axilla, the note may more resonant than other areas. Lesions which are deep-seated (>5 cm from the chest wall) and smaller lesion (<3 cm in diameter) may not alter percussion note but visible on the X-ray.
- *Abnormal resonant note*:
  - Myotatic irritability (percussion myokymia)—in case of emaciation or wasting of the patient, a percussion stroke over the front of the chest wall produces fibrillatory contraction of the muscle but no note is produced.
  - Hyperresonant note—is obtained when the airspace in the lung contains more air than normal. It is seen in pneumothorax, emphysema (usually bilateral hyperresonance), compensatory emphysema (unilateral), or a large superficial cavity or emphysematous bulla.

- Tympanitic note—drum-like note normally heard over stomach and intestines. In the chest, this note may be heard in diaphragmatic hernia.
- Subtympanitic note (Skodaic resonance)—hyper-resonant note with boxy quality just above the level of pleural effusion. This is produced because of the relaxed lung partially filled with air that is pushed upward and toward the hilum.
- Impaired note—when a part of the lung has no air or less air, it fails to vibrate sufficiently on percussion with slight loss of resonance and called impaired note as it happens in consolidation or collapse.
- Dull note—inflammation of lung parenchyma results in collection of fluid, exudates, and infiltration of cells in alveoli as in consolidation, which will reduce the resonant note and more muffled than the impaired note. Also, it can occur in lung collapse, large tumors, and thickened pleura.
- Stony dull—the best example is pleural effusion because when examiner percusses over the chest wall practically, no sound is heard as if percussing over the thighs or over a stone. Dampening note is due to change in the interphase (the fluid dampens the conduction of vibration to chest wall). But in a pleural effusion above the fluid level, it may be resonant note or subtympanitic note because of collapsed lung. It can also occur in solid tumor.
- Cracked pot resonance—may be demonstrated over a cavity communicating with a bronchus. It occurs when the patient coughs, the air is expelled, and examiner may obtain a tympanitic-like resonance.

Tidal Percussion

Percussion to find out the lower border of lung resonance on each side on deep inspiration and expiration. This will help in finding out the diaphragmatic movement. This can be done either anteriorly or posteriorly.

S-shaped Curve of Ellis

This is useful to find the upper extent of pleural fluid (which is highest in the axilla and lowest in the spine assuming the shape of letter "S"). Some authors attribute this to capillary suction. In a moderate effusion, lung collapses toward hilum to give space to the fluid to rise in the axilla and this can differentiate hydropneumothorax and encysted effusion where the fluid does not go higher up in the axilla.

Start in front where the stony dullness is present and then go laterally and the examiner has to percuss the extent of dullness in the axilla and then come posteriorly where the dullness is felt. In uncomplicated pleural effusion, where the fluid is free, the stony dull note will be higher up in the axilla indicating the fluid is at a higher level.

Straight Line Dullness

It is one of the key points in diagnosing hydropneumothorax and pyopneumothorax. The percussion note does not go up the axilla, but the dullness can be elicited as a straight line around the hemithorax and above the dull note there will be hyperresonant note because of air. Other two clinical features for diagnosing hydropneumothorax and pyopneumothorax are shifting dullness and succussion splash (on auscultation).

Shifting Dullness

Percussion for shifting dullness

Useful in hydropneumothorax and also to detect small pleural effusion. When there is air and fluid, the fluid shifts to dependent position and the lung and air float up. The patient is asked to lie down or sit down and start percussing from above down. In the upper part, hyperresonant note may be heard and below where the fluid is present, there is stony dullness. Now turn the patient to lateral decubitus position (if the lesion is on right side, ask the patient to lie on left) and wait for sometime before percussion. Now percussion is done and the dull area becomes resonant because the fluid has shifted. Shifting dullness may be absent in pleural effusion. If the examiner suspects pyothorax, the patient has to lie on the lateral side for about 5 minutes or more because the thick pus takes sometime to move unlike the pleural fluid.

Cardiac Dullness

Along with palpation by percussion, cardiac dullness can be elicited.

- *Percussion of left heart border*: Ask the patient to lie supine and locate the 5th intercostal space on the left side from the sternal angle. Percuss from midsternal line (usually dull) parallel to the lateral sternal border and percuss till resonant note heard. This is the left border of heart. If the distance between dull note and resonant note is >11 cm, it may indicate cardiomegaly.
- *Percussion of right heart border*: As above patient is to be in supine position. By percussing along the midclavicular line, locate the upper border of liver. Percuss parallel along the right lateral sternal margin and find out the area of dullness. Right heart is enlarged, if the dull note is >1 cm from the lateral sternal border.

Liver Dullness

Percuss anteriorly on the right side from infraclavicular area in the midclavicular line and anterior axillary line and normal liver dullness is heard in the 5th or 6th intercostal space position.

Splenic Dullness

Small area of dullness can be demonstrated in the 8th intercostal space in midaxillary line on the left side due to the presence of spleen.

Grocco's Triangle

It is in the form of a triangle bounded medially by midspinal line to the level of 10th thoracic vertebra (lower border of lung resonance), below by horizontal lining extending outward from 10th thoracic vertebra for about 3-7 cm and laterally by a curved line connecting the above lines. This area may be obliterated in presence of moderate-to-large pleural effusion over the back of the chest on the contralateral side. This may be due to displacement of posterior mediastinum to the opposite side as a result of fluid collection.

Garland's Triangle

Roughly, a triangular area where tympanitic note or Skodaic resonance is heard in pleural effusion because of the relaxed lung above.

Traube's Space

Semilunar space, bounded by pulmonary resonance, on the right by liver dullness, on the left by splenic dullness, and below by the left costal margin overlies the stomach contents.

Auscultation

There is variation in airflow in larger airways which is turbulent flow whereas it becomes laminar in smaller airways. The noise of the flow varies from 200 to 2,000 Hz and when air reaches the smaller airways and alveoli, filtration takes place and the sound becomes softer (200-400 Hz) and conducted to the chest wall as normal breath sounds previously termed as "vesicular".

The intensity of breath heard through the chest wall depends on the rate of air flow and the acoustic properties of lung and chest wall. In consolidation, there is no filtration of air by the alveoli and directly conducted to chest wall and the sound heard is similar to that heard over the trachea (tubular breathing), when the sound is reflected at the interface between the lung and any other media such as air (pneumothorax) or fluid (pleural effusion).

Auscultation of the lungs includes breath sounds, its character and intensity, vocal resonance, and adventitious sounds.

Principles of Auscultation

- Auscultation should be done in a quiet room, preferably in a sitting position. If the patient cannot assume sitting posture, roll the patient from one side to the other to examine the back.
- Ask the patient to take deep breaths through the open mouth.
- Using the diaphragm of the stethoscope, start auscultation anteriorly at the apices and move downward till no breath sound is appreciated. Next, listen to the back, starting at the apices, and moving downward. At least one complete respiratory cycle should be heard at each site.
- Always compare symmetrical points on each side.
- Listen for the quality of the breath sounds, the intensity of the breath sounds, and the presence of adventitious sounds.

The examiner has to listen for both inspiratory and expiratory breath sounds in all the topographical areas as described earlier.

Listen carefully for intensity, quality, comparison of inspiratory and expiratory breath sounds, and prolongation of breath sounds.

In this book, the authors confine to two types of breath sounds for easy understanding:
1. Normal breath sound (vesicular breath sound).
2. *Bronchial breathing of three types*:
    i. Tubular breathing
    ii. Cavernous breathing
    iii. Amphoric breathing

Vesicular Breath Sound

Vesicular breath sound is a misnomer as vesicles means alveoli and this gives the impression that the breath sound is originating at the alveolar level. However, breath sounds cannot be generated at the alveolar level since airflow is laminar within the alveoli. The expiratory sound is audible only in the early phase. The short expiratory phase is due to the passive nature of expiration resulting in generation of less turbulent airflow. The origin of both phases of respiration is also in different sites. The inspiratory component originates in the lobar and segmental airways whereas the expiratory component arises from more central airways.

Characteristics of normal breath sound (**Fig. 20**) are as follows:
- Rustling of leaves during breeze.
- Inspiratory sound is louder and greater in intensity than expiratory sound.
- Longer duration of inspiratory sound ratio of 3:1.
- Absence of pause between inspiration and expiration.

If any change in the normal breath sound is examined, the examiner has to think about an underlying pathology.

Bronchial Breath Sounds

Characteristics of bronchial breath sound (**Fig. 21**) are as follows:

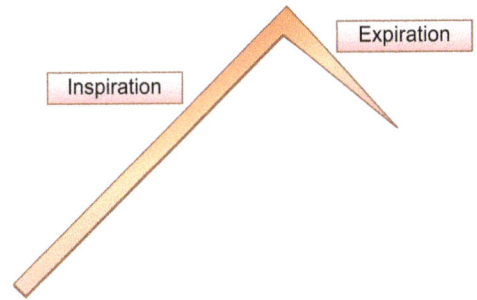

FIG. 20: Normal breath sound.

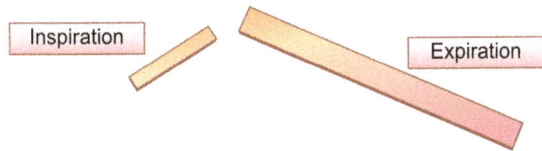

FIG. 21: Bronchial breath sounds.

- Expiratory component is louder and longer than inspiratory component.
- The ratio between inspiratory and expiratory sound is 2:3.
- There is a pause between inspiratory and expiratory sound.

Tubular: Normal heard over trachea and this can be kept as reference point to make out whether it is tubular or normal breath sound. Tubular breathing is high-pitched in quality heard over consolidation, any mass overlying major airways, above pleural effusion, and upper lobe fibrosis.

Cavernous: Low-pitched hollow quality usually heard over thick-walled cavity and "pulled trachea syndrome". The cavity should be >3 cm in diameter and <5 cm from chest wall.

Amphoric: High-pitched bronchial breathing with metallic quality and it resembles blowing through a narrow metal pipe in thin-walled cavity communicating with bronchus, bronchopleural fistula. The presence of amphoric breathing is pathognomonic in diagnosis of bronchopleural fistula.

Adventitious/Added Sounds

Adventitious sounds are additional respiratory sounds superimposed on normal breath sounds. Adventitious lung sounds are classified into two main categories: (1) Continuous and; (2) Interrupted sounds. Interrupted or discontinuous sounds are further classified into fine and coarse crackles and continuous sounds are further classified into wheeze and rhonchi (International Lung Sound Association).

Wheeze and Rhonchi

Wheeze and rhonchi are continuous musical lung sounds. Continuous adventitious sound lasts >250 ms. The American Thoracic Society (ATS) Committee on pulmonary nomenclature defines wheeze as high-pitched continuous sounds with a dominant frequency of 400 Hz or more and rhonchi as low-pitched continuous musical sounds with a dominant frequency of about 200 Hz or less.

The mechanisms of wheeze are:
- Narrowing of airways.
- Mucosal edema
- Mucus plugging
  It is also produced by vibration of opposing airways.

Monophonic wheeze: Single musical note of constant pitch timing and site during inspiration. The monophonic wheeze may better heard (higher) during expiration than inspiration, probably due to tightness of stenosis, foreign body, malignancies, and intramural and extramural compression (e.g., lymph node or mass obstructing the bronchus).

Polyphonic wheeze: It is an expiratory musical sound containing several notes at different pitch throughout expiration as in asthma and chronic bronchitis.

Stridor occurs in both phases of respiration. It is due to narrowing of trachea or larynx.

Crackles (Rales, Crepitations)

Crackles are discontinuous, explosive, and nonmusical adventitious lung sounds normally heard in inspiration and sometimes during expiration. Crackles are usually classified as fine and coarse crackles based on their duration, loudness, pitch, timing in the respiratory cycle, and relationship to coughing and changing body position.

Mechanisms of the production of crackles: Initially, production of crackles was attributed to the passage of air through the accumulated secretions within the large and medium size airways, creating the bubbling sounds.

Forgacs proposed the second theory of crackles. According to Forgacs, small airways that were collapsed during expiration snap open during inspiration as a gradient of gas pressure is developed across the collapsed airways. Sudden explosive opening of the collapsed airways induces a rapid equalization of gas pressures resulting in oscillations of the gas column and development of crackles.

Stress Relaxation Quadrupole Hypothesis

Fredberg and Holford proposed the stress relaxation quadrupole hypothesis of crackles generation. According to this hypothesis, crackles are produced by the vibration in the walls of small airways and not by the air column within airways. Crackles arise due to the sudden opening and closing of airways, resulting in stress waves propagation in the lung parenchyma.

Liquid Bridge Hypothesis

Liquid bridges are formed due to abnormal mechanical instabilities in the small airways. Liquid bridge ruptures are responsible for the inspiratory crackle sound and formation of the liquid bridge explains the expiratory crackle.

- *Early inspiratory crackles*: Chronic bronchitis, stage of resolution of pneumonia probably because of reopening of more proximal airways.
- *Midinspiratory crackles*: Bronchiectasis, midinspiratory phase is represented from segmental bronchi to terminal bronchioles. They are audible at the mouth and no postural variation and may be altered by coughing. The character may be leathery.
- *Late inspiratory crackles*: Interstitial lung diseases and pulmonary edema. Usually heard at the bases. They are produced at small airways. It is due to explosive reopening during the latter part of inspiration of small distal airways with abnormally opposed walls during the previous expiration. They are not conducted to the mouth and changes with posture. They are called "Velcro" crackles. Leaning forward will reduce the intensity of the crackles in diffuse parenchymal lung disease, but in pulmonary edema as it takes longer time for the fluid to shift.

Pulmonary Squeak

It follows an inspiratory crackle and probably caused by vibration in the wall of a bronchiole as it opens following abnormal closure. It may be heard in diffuse parenchymal lung disease and hypersensitivity pneumonitis.

Vocal Resonance

The mechanism is same as vocal fremitus.

Usually, low frequency is transmitted to chest wall after it gets filtered by alveoli in a normal subject. In certain diseases, it may alter.

The sound produced in larynx is transmitted to chest wall as vibration and the patient is asked to say some number in their language (usually one...one...one) which should be distinct and patient is asked to repeat it when the examiner places the diaphragm of the stethoscope on the chest wall. The spoken words should be clear and with the same intensity.

The words the patient uttered are conducted to the chest wall and it will be weak and muffled in normal individuals. The examiner has to compare symmetrical areas starting from supraclavicular to mammary areas, axillary and infra-axillary areas, and posteriorly suprascapular, interscapular, and infrascapular areas.

Vocal resonance is increased in consolidation, fibrosis and reduced in pleural effusion, pneumothorax, and lung collapse.

Pleural Rub

Pleural rub is rubbing, grating, and leathery sound. It is usually localized and has loud intensity, superficial in character, and the sound is intensified when the stethoscope is pressed over the area.

There is a thin layer of lubricating fluid separating parietal pleura from the visceral pleura in a healthy individual. But in inflammation of pleura, the inflamed surfaces rub each other because of the lack of lubricating fluid which produces both pain and friction in a localized area. It is commonly heard in the infra-axillary area but rarely diffuse in nature. Pleural rub is usually heard at the end of inspiration (when the two surfaces rub each other) and at the beginning of expiration when the two layers are in close approximation. Unlike crackles, the rub is not altered with coughing.

It can be differentiated from pericardial rub which is continuous whereas pleural rub is absent when the patient is asked to stop breathing.

Succussion Splash

It is a common sign in hydropneumothorax, pyopneumothorax, and hemopneumothorax, i.e., when there is air and fluid in the pleural space, succussion splash can be appreciated. Keep the diaphragm of the stethoscope over the fluid-air interphase and shake the patient vigorously. If the sign is positive, a splashing sound is heard. This can be also heard over a large cavity containing fluid and air in the lung and also in herniation of stomach or colon into thoracic cavity through diaphragm. For a clinical diagnosis of hydropneumothorax or pyopneumothorax, the three important signs are: On percussion—shifting dullness, straight line dullness and on auscultation—succussion splash. The sign can be reproduced by the following method—take a bottle containing water which is half full and the examiner can appreciate the three signs. Succussion splash can be heard by shaking the bottle.

Hamman Sign or Mediastinal Crunch

It may be heard in case of left-sided pneumothorax. It is a crunching sound heard when there is movement of air during the systolic contraction of the heart. This also can occur in pneumomediastinum, bullous emphysema of the lingular lobe, dilatation of stomach, dilatation of the lower third of esophagus, and pneumoperitoneum with the rise in the left diaphragm.

Post-tussive Suction

It is heard over a thin-walled large cavity in communication with the bronchus. Ask the patient to cough and the air in the cavity will be emptied out, now keep the diaphragm of the stethoscope over the cavity and ask the patient to inspire and the examiner will hear a gushing sound as if air being sucked into the cavity.

Bronchophony

When spoken sounds become more loud or intense and close to the ear while auscultation, it is called bronchophony. It occurs in consolidation above the level of pleural effusion, lung cavity located superficially. This is due to conduction of the sound directly to the chest wall without filtration taking place in the lung.

Whispering Pectoriloquy

To elicit whispering pectoriloquy, the patient is asked to whisper syllables and this may be heard through the stethoscope very clearly as in cavity with communication with the bronchus, consolidation, compressed lung above pleural effusion, and obstruction of large bronchus by a tumor proximal to the site of obstruction.

Aegophony/EA sign

Previously, the sounds heard were described as bleating of a goat. The patient is asked to say "Eee" and examiner will hear it as "aa" through the stethoscope. It can be appreciated just above the pleural effusion and consolidation.

Coin Test

A coin is placed in the interscapular area and assistant taps the coin with another coin and the examiner auscultates in the anterior chest wall. In case of pneumothorax, a bell-like sound will be heard by the examiner and is called bell tympany.

Scratch Sign

The diaphragm of the stethoscope is placed over the sternum. The skin of the patient is scratched at equidistant points from the stethoscope. In pneumothorax, the sound heard will be louder when comparing with the normal side. This is due to high frequency of sound absorption by the adjacent normal lung.

d'Espine Sign

Whispered voice heard in the normal individuals over the spines of lower cervical vertebra. But in infancy and childhood, it can be heard below the 7th cervical vertebra and at the level of 3rd thoracic vertebra in adults. When whispered voice is heard below these levels, d'Espine sign is positive. A positive d'Espine sign may be suggestive of enlarged mediastinal or tracheobronchial lymph nodes, tumor in the posterior mediastinum, or in central pneumonia.

CHAPTER 4

Common Investigations in Respiratory Evaluation

INTRODUCTION

The main aim of supporting and relevant investigations is to confirm the diagnosis we have already made from detailed history taking and clinical examination.

At present day scenario, we have to depend more on these investigations, in case if there is medical litigation to protect ourselves. In a tertiary care center, opinion can be sought from other specialty departments, e.g., cardiothoracic surgery, ear, nose, and throat (ENT), etc. Various strains and culture methods are available in microbiology to identify various pathogens. In pathology also, various strains are used. The main investigation support is from the radiology department for confirming various diagnoses.

As medical tests are becoming exorbitantly expensive, basic and cost-effective investigations should be ordered. In future, more supportive tests may be available.

DIAGNOSTIC TESTS

- *Blood routine*—hemoglobin, total leukocyte count, differential count (especially eosinophils, lymphocytes), erythrocyte sedimentation rate (ESR), tests for human

immunodeficiency virus (HIV) (if history of high-risk behavior), and also in all presumptive tuberculosis (TB) patients.
- *Sputum collection*—by expectoration, laryngeal swabs, gastric aspiration, pharyngeal or tonsillar swabs, tracheobronchial aspiration, bronchoalveolar lavage (BAL), and induced sputum through inhaled mucolytics (if difficult to expectorate due to thick viscid sputum).

  With the sputum, following tests can be performed:
  - Acid-fast bacilli (AFB) staining—two samples; direct smear by Ziehl–Neelsen (ZN) stain, light-emitting diode (LED) microscope, cartridge-based nucleic acid amplification test (CBNAAT), and line probe assay (LPA).
  - Acid-fast bacilli culture and sensitivity—if drug resistance suspected along with the other modern techniques [e.g., polymerase chain reaction (PCR)].
  - In bacterial infections—culture and sensitivity
  - Fungal hyphae, fungal staining, and culture
  - Bronchial asthma—eosinophils, plugs, casts, creola bodies, Curschmann's spirals, and Charcot–Leyden crystals [also in allergic bronchopulmonary aspergillosis (ABPA)].
  - Asbestos bodies—asbestosis
  - Hooklets—hydatid cyst, entamoeba histolytica—hepatopulmonary amebiasis
  - Sputum malignant cytology—carcinoma bronchus
- Urine examination tests for COVID-19 (if indicated).
- *Tests for COVID-19*—commonly performed tests for antigen detection in India - Nasopharyngeal or throat swab and RT-PCR. More tests are being tried.
- X-ray of chest [preferably posteroanterior (PA) view or anteroposterior (AP), lateral, lateral decubitus, lordotic view, etc., as the condition demands].

- Ultrasonography (USG) (thorax and abdomen)
- Fasting and postprandial blood sugar (FBS and PPBS)—preferably for all the patients above the age of 30 years.
- Paracentesis thoracis in pleural effusion (with all relevant investigations).
- Pleural biopsy
- Lymph node—fine-needle aspiration cytology (FNAC) and biopsy.
- Liver function testing (LFT)—if indicated.
- Renal function testing (RFT)—if indicated.
- Pulmonary function testing (PFT) [spirometry, diffusing capacity of the lungs for carbon monoxide (DLCO), and body plethysmography].
- Peak flow meter—measure peak expiratory flow rate.
- Electrocardiogram (ECG) and echocardiogram
- Computed tomography—high-resolution computed tomography (HRCT) or with contrast as the situation demands.
- Arterial blood gas (ABG)
- Tuberculin testing—mantoux test (indicates tuberculous infection and not the disease).
- Other diagnostic skin testing—hydatid, sarcoidosis, histoplasmosis, blastomycosis, etc.
- Allergy testing—intradermal and sublingual immunotherapy (SLIT)
- Magnetic resonance imaging (MRI)—if necessary.
- Barium swallow—in case of dysphagia, but it can be visualized in CT.
- Bronchoscopy—rigid and fiberoptic bronchoscopy: BAL, biopsy, bronchial brushing, transbronchial biopsy, and transbronchial needle aspiration.
- Endobronchial ultrasound (EBUS)
- Percutaneous or open lung biopsy

- Immunological tests, if indicated—immunoglobulin G (IgG), immunoglobulin M (IgM), and immunoglobulin E (IgE).
- Pleuroscopy
- Video-assisted thoracoscopy (VATS)
- Mediastinoscopy (not popular now)
- Pulmonary angiography
- Ventilation-perfusion scan
- Positron emission tomography (PET) scan
- Polysomnography for sleep-related breathing disorders.
- *Inflammometry:* Fractional exhaled nitric oxide (FeNO) (bronchial asthma, cystic fibrosis, and primary ciliary dyskinetic syndromes) and exhaled breath condensate analysis.
- Transmission electron microscopy (TEM)—primary ciliary dyskinesia.

CERTAIN IMPORTANT TESTS (NOT COMMONLY DONE) (TABLE 1)

TABLE 1: Certain important tests (Not commonly done).

Suspected condition	Suggested test
Pulmonary embolism	D-dimer
Inherited emphysema	α1-antitrypsin
Cystic fibrosis	Specific genetic tests
Lung cancer	Tumor markers (CEA and SCC)
Malignant mesothelioma (mesothelin and fibrillin)	Tumor markers
Pneumonia	Serum procalcitonin
Latent tuberculosis infection	IGRAs
Sarcoidosis	SACE and serum calcium levels
Hypersensitive pneumonitis	Specific precipitating antibodies

Continued

Continued

Suspected condition	Suggested test
Connective tissue disorders	Rheumatoid factor, ANA, etc.
Unexplained dyspnea (to rule out cardiac cause)	NT-proBNP—increase in heart failure.

(ANA: antinuclear antibody; CEA: carcinoembryonic antigen; SACE: serum angiotensin-converting enzyme; SCC: squamous cell carcinoma; NT- proBNP: N-terminal pro-brain natriuretic peptide; IGRAs: Interferon-gamma release assays)

Now that we have done the physical examination, we will get back to the three sample case studies illustrated in Chapter 2 and try to come to a diagnosis.

CASE STUDY 1

General Examination
- On general examination, there was no pallor, icterus, lymphadenopathy, and pedal edema. Clubbing grade 2 was present and body mass index (BMI) was 18 kg/m^2.
- *Upper respiratory tract:* Normal
- *Lower respiratory tract:* Trachea and apex beat appear shifted showing mediastinal shift on inspection.
- *Palpation:* Movements reduced with reduction in chest expansion in the right infraclavicular area. Vocal fremitus was increased in the above area.
- *Percussion:* Note impaired.
- *Auscultation:* Bronchial breathing was present with coarse crackles with absence of wheeze. Vocal resonance was increased.

Provisional diagnosis from history and examination can be:
- Pulmonary tuberculosis (can be reactivation or fibrosis of right upper lobe).

- Bronchogenic carcinoma (smoker and scar carcinoma).
- Bronchiectasis

To come to a final diagnosis, following investigations can be done:
- Blood—hemoglobin, total count—differential blood count, and ESR.
- Fasting blood sugar and PPBS (considering the age factor and suspicion of pulmonary TB).
- Sputum for AFB for 2 days.
- Sputum culture and sensitivity (especially in bronchiectasis).
- X-ray of chest—posterior-anterior view.
- High-resolution computed tomography to rule out bronchiectasis and malignancy.
- Fiberoptic bronchoscopy in case of malignancy.

If sputum is positive for AFB, then invasive or expensive investigations can be avoided.

CASE STUDY 2

- *On general examination:* Clubbing was present (grade 3) and BMI was 22 kg/m^2.
- *Inspection:* Tracheal shift to left and apex beat shifted 2 inches lateral to the midclavicular line toward the axilla.
- *On palpation:* Increased vocal fremitus on the left supraclavicular and infraclavicular areas.
- *Percussion:* Impaired note in the above areas.
- *Auscultation:* Bronchial breathing in the above areas, but normal breath sounds in other areas. Crackles were heard over the left supraclavicular and infraclavicular areas which are conducted to the mouth.

All the earlier mentioned differential diagnoses (page no. 35) may be applicable in this case. So, the battery of laboratory investigations may be extensive.

Investigations

- Blood—hemoglobin, total count—differential blood count, and ESR.
- Fasting blood sugar and PPBS (considering the age factor and suspicion of pulmonary TB).
- Sputum for AFB for 2 days (if sputum is negative for AFB), the following tests to be done:
  - Sputum culture and sensitivity (especially in bronchiectasis).
- X-ray of chest—posterior-anterior view
- Liver function test
- High-resolution computed tomography to rule out bronchiectasis and malignancy.
- Spirometry
- Fiberoptic bronchoscopy in case of malignancy.

CASE STUDY 3

- Patient was tachypneic with accessory muscles acting, but cooperative in giving detailed history. No cyanosis or dehydration and oxygen saturation (SpO_2) was 96%.
- *Percussion:* Bilateral hyper-resonant note.
- *Auscultation:* Normal breath sounds with bilateral wheeze. Probable diagnosis—acute severe asthma probably exacerbated by secondary infection.
- Patient has to be nebulized immediately and intravenous (IV) steroids may be given (detailed treatment of asthma is given later).

When the patient improves, following investigations should be done:
- X-ray of chest—posterior-anterior view
- Blood—hemoglobin, total count—differential blood count, and ESR.

- Fasting blood sugar and PPBS (family history of diabetes mellitus and probably prolonged steroid intake).
- Sputum for AFB for 2 days.
- Sputum culture and sensitivity
- Once the patient settles, spirometry can be done, if sputum for AFB is negative.

CHAPTER 5

Roentgenography: "A Step-by-step Approach to Reading of Chest X-ray"

INTRODUCTION

Reading an X-ray correctly requires some expertise which you gain over years and after seeing multitude of X-rays. Overreading or underreading may lead to disastrous results, especially when you are the final say as a pulmonologist or physician and may cause unnecessary financial burden and mental agony to the patient.

Although imaging examinations are valuable in the study of intrathoracic disease, they do not supplement the importance of a thorough history and physical examination. In addition, blood tests, diagnostic skin tests, sputum cultures, biopsy, and especially bronchoscopy have the ability to add a unique information perspective for diagnosing a case. The clinician is cautioned to recognize the limitations of imaging and the unique benefits provided by other diagnostic studies. Serial X-ray of the patient is useful to avoid unnecessary investigations [such as old fibrosis, solitary pulmonary nodule (SPN) which is static over years, etc.].

The authors are in the process of bringing out a Handbook on Radiological Approach to Respiratory Medicine to help in understanding chest X-rays (CXRs) and interpreting them with confidence.

The standard radiographic examination of the chest consists:
- Posteroanterior (PA) view—most common

Certain other views may be helpful for better understanding:
- Anteroposterior (AP) view
- Right or left lateral view/projection
- Oblique view
- Lateral decubitus view
- Lordotic view
- Apicogram
- Penetrated view

Procedure: Chest radiography uses high peak kilovoltage (110–150 kVp) exposures during full patient inspiratory effort.

POSTEROANTERIOR VIEW

Commonly prefered to visualize the lung fields better unless the patient is very sick to stand, in supine position, or using a bedside portable X-ray machine.

In PA view, the cartridge is kept in contact with the anterior chest wall and the X-ray tube is 6 feet (2 m) behind the subject. In this view, the subject stands erect with the hands on the hip with bent elbows and made to hold the breath after deep inspiration. A perfect X-ray should include the neck and upper abdomen. While reading the X-ray, the reader preferably should be 6 feet (2 m) from the X-ray lobby (X-ray viewer). This will be enable the reader to clearly visualize the lung fields and heart contour (heart shadow approximately to the actual size). In PA view, X-ray beams traverse the subject from posterior to anterior and strike the film.

ANTEROPOSTERIOR VIEW

Not commonly employed for reading lung fields because of poor orientation; usually, such X-rays are available in intensive care unit (ICU) when the patient is sick or unable to stand using a bedside portable X-ray machine. AP view positioning of cartridge and subject's position is exactly opposite to PA view. Here, the cartridge is kept in contact with the posterior chest wall and the X-ray tube is 6 feet (2 m) in front of the subject. In AP view, X-ray beams traverse the subject from anterior to posterior before striking the film (**Table 1**).

LATERAL VIEW OF X-RAY (RIGHT LATERAL AND LEFT LATERAL)

In the lateral view also, the subject will be standing 6 feet (2 m) away from the tube. Subject's right side is against the cartridge in right lateral and in left lateral, left side of the subject is placed against the cartridge. In viewing the right lateral film, the anterior wall of the X-ray corresponds to the reader's right side and for left lateral film, the anterior wall of the X-ray corresponds to the viewer's left side (**Fig. 3**). Anatomical features such as liver, domes of diaphragm,

TABLE 1: Major differences between PA and AP view.

PA view (Fig. 1)	AP view (Fig. 2)
Scapula in periphery	Scapula over lung fields
Clavicles project over lung fields	Clavicles are above the apex of lung fields
Posterior ribs are distinct	Anterior ribs are distinct
Cardiac shadow is normal without cardiac pathology	Cardiac shadow is larger (magnification)

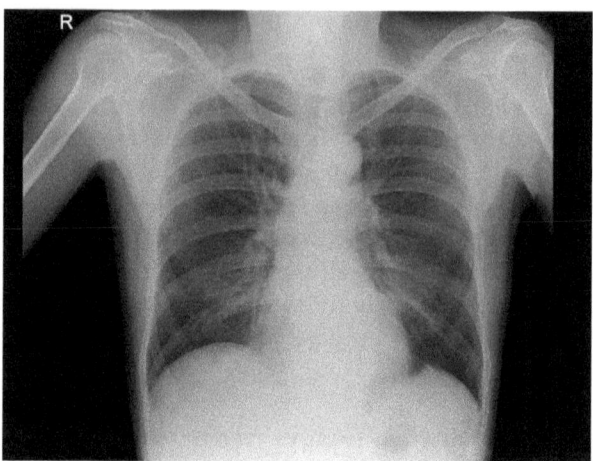

FIG. 1: Chest X-ray standard posteroanterior (PA) view.

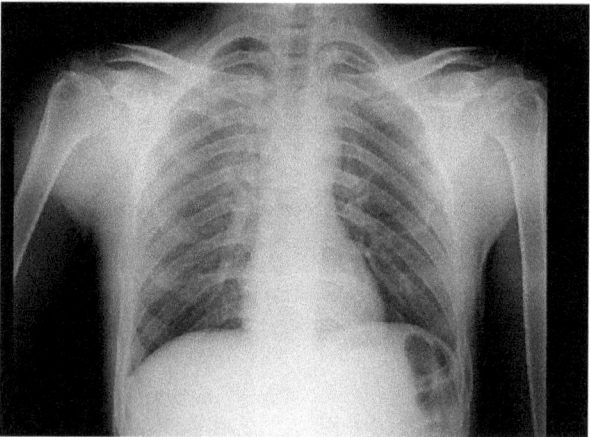

FIG. 2: Chest X-ray standard anteroposterior (AP) view.

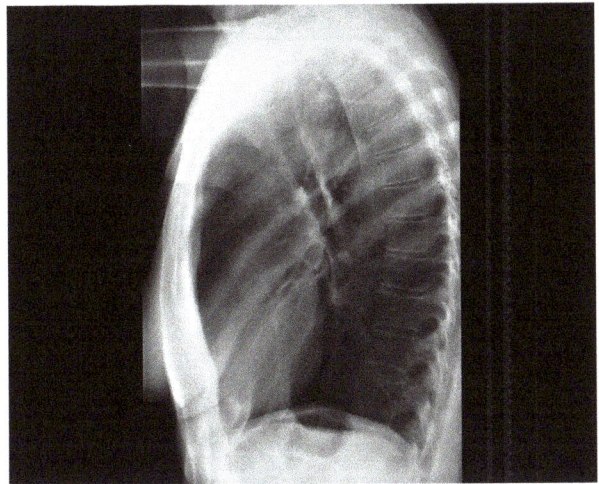

FIG. 3: Chest X-ray lateral view (left lateral).

interlobar fissures, and fundal gas can be seen under the left diaphragm (cystic fibrosis, situs inversus). Lateral views also help in localization of an opacity—anteriorly placed or posteriorly placed and give a clear picture of the retrosternal space (emphysema).

LATERAL DECUBITUS VIEW (FIG. 4)

Subject lying on the side (right or left depending on the pathology). Helpful in demonstrating a small pneumothorax or pleural effusion.

LORDOTIC VIEW (FIG. 5)

The beam is angled up toward head and the orientation appears different. The clavicles will project superiorly relative

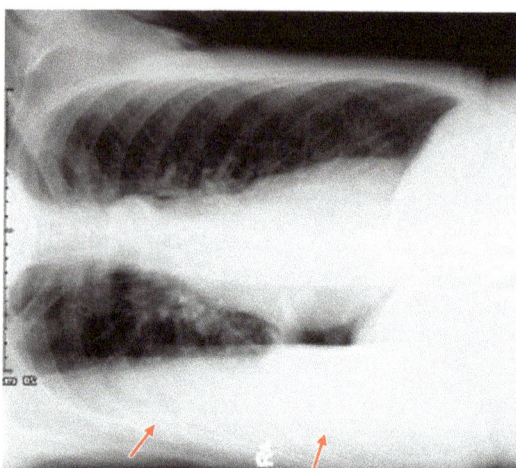

FIG. 4: Chest X-ray right lateral decubitus film showing right pleural effusion (red arrows).

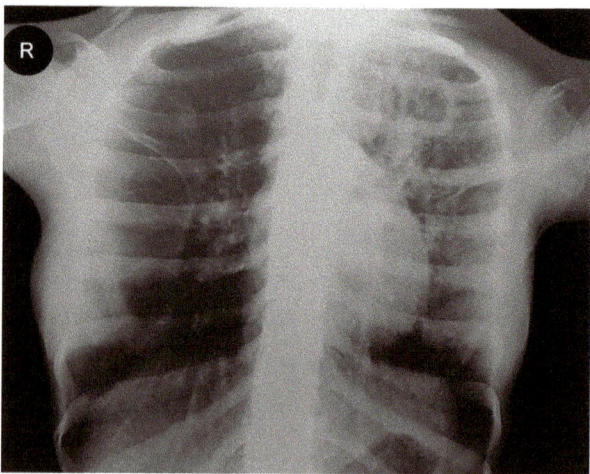

FIG. 5: Lordotic view or apicogram showing a well-defined cavity over left lung apex.

to the upper thorax and cause distortion of mediastinal anatomy. Ribs assume more horizontal position. The reader will be able to clearly visualize the thoracic apex (inlet). Hence, this view is also called as "Apicogram".

OBLIQUE VIEW (FIG. 6)

Helpful in localizing lesion, visualizing its borders, and in projecting it free of overlying structures. In bilateral pulmonary disesase, this view is preferred to lateral view (with the advent of CT, its role is not frequently employed).

COMMON TERMS

- Black—air/gas—radiolucency (translucency)
- White-fluid/fat/solid structures—radiopacity (opacity)

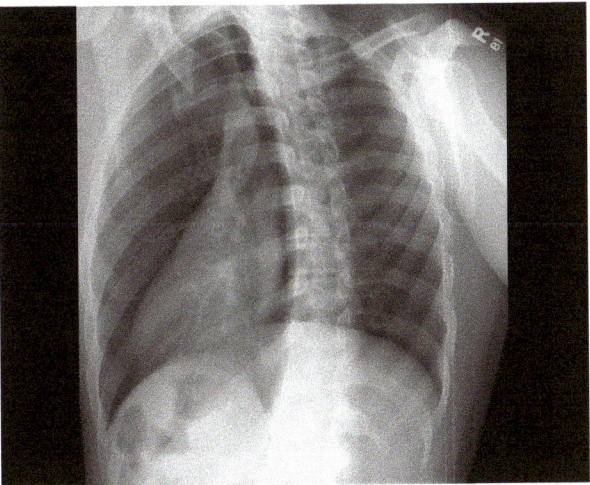

FIG. 6: Chest X-ray oblique view.

SYSTEMATIC READING OF CHEST X-RAY

Always check the following:
- Name of patient
- Age
- Sex
- Side marked on X-ray (right or left)—orientation
- Hospital number with date
- Projection (PA or AP, lateral decubitus, lordotic, penetrated, and apicogram)
- Supine/portable—AP (mainly ICU X-rays)

Rule Out Artifacts (Fig. 7)

Once all the above details are noted, in case of any doubt, the patient may be taken to the radiology department for clarification or may have to take a fresh X-ray.

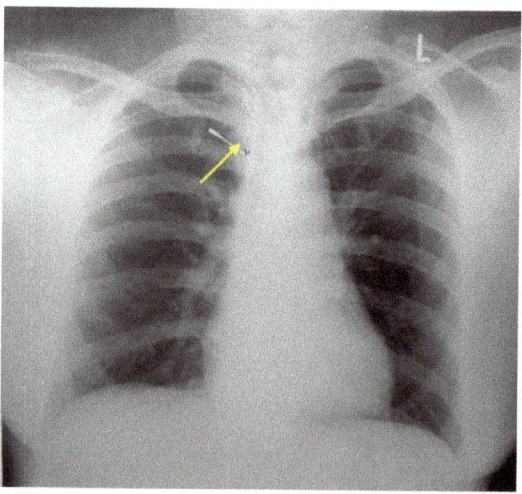

FIG. 7: Chest X-ray showing radiodensity in right upper lobe due to artifact (safety pin) (yellow arrow).

Systematic Reading of Chest X-ray (Posteroanterior View)

Technical Compatibility for Reading

Phase of Breathing, Positioning, and Penetration

- The radiograph should display the entire thorax (preferably neck and upper abdomen included).
- Good patient inspiratory result is noted by observing the posterior portions of the first ten ribs (or anterior portions of the first seven ribs) above the right hemidiaphragm. Commonly, the right hemidiaphragm is used as a reference point (situs inversus—should be remembered) because the position of the left hemidiaphragm is more variable due to the subjacent gastric air bubble.
- Heart shadow should be clearly seen. In a properly exposed film, both costophrenic angle and lung apices can be clearly seen. Spines of the vertebrae are barely seen through the cardiac shadow.
- Diagnostic purposes sometimes warrant taking films during patient expiration. For instance, if a "check-valve" bronchial obstruction is present, the involved lung demonstrates a pathologic state in which it remains well-inflated on an expiration film.

Penetration (normal)

- Should see ribs and vertebral bodies through the heart.
- Barely see the intervertebral disk through the heart.
- Should see pulmonary vessels near the edges of lung.
- These are clearly seen in overpenetrated films but not in underpenetrated films.

Overpenetrated film (**Fig. 8**):
- Hyperlucency (lung fields appear dark).
- Can visualize spine well beyond diaphragm.
- Inadequate clarity of lung fields.

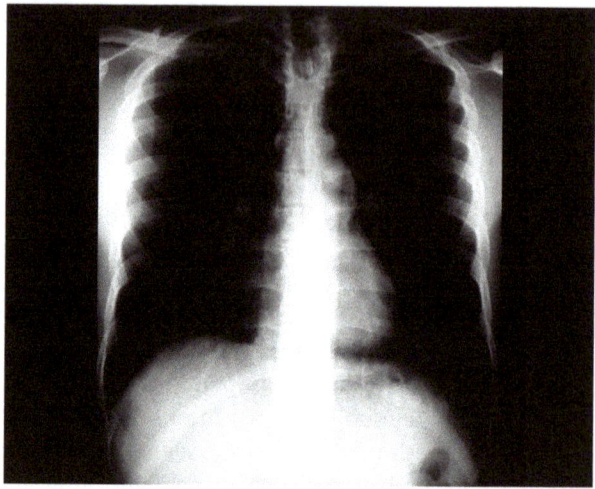

FIG. 8: Overpenetrated chest X-ray showing dark lung fields.

Underpenetrated film (**Fig. 9**):
- Hemidiaphragms are obscured.
- Pulmonary markings appear more prominent.

Position of the Subject

In a well-positioned film, the medial ends of the clavicles should be equidistant from the spine of vertebra. If the film is rotated, the reader may interpret wrongly—hilum may look more prominent on one side, misinterpretation of vascular markings, etc. (**Fig. 10**).

Reading of Chest X-ray

Read from outward to inward: Systematic reading.

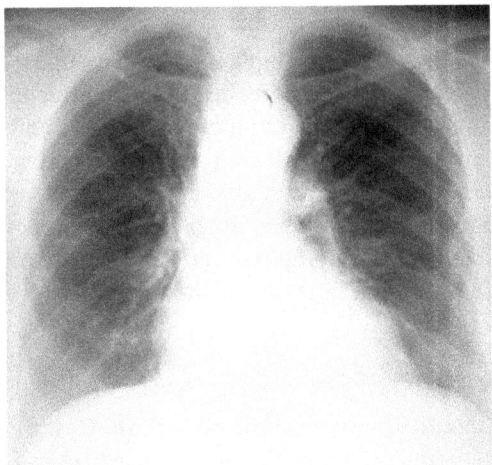

FIG. 9: Underpenetrated chest X-ray showing prominence of lung markings.

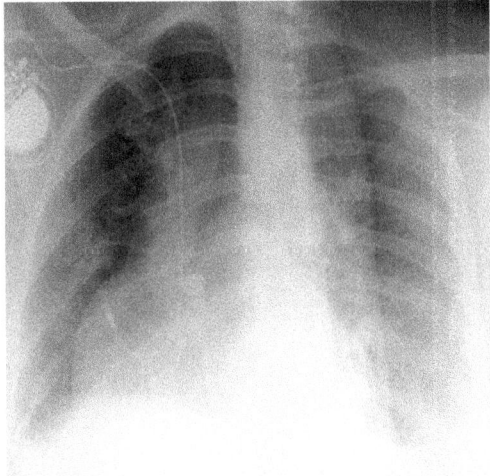

FIG. 10: Grossly rotated film showing mediastinal shift to right.

Soft Tissue

Normal shadows—breast, nipple shadow may appear as round opacities usually in the fourth or lower anterior intercostal space usually bilateral and symmetrical (**Figs. 11** and **12**).

Abnormal shadows—pleated hair in females causing opacity such as shadow in the apical region, intercostal drainage tube, lipomas, subcutaneous calcifications (**Figs. 13** and **14**), subcutaneous emphysema (**Fig. 15**), sebaceous cyst, or any other swelling can cast a shadow on PA view (**Figs. 16A** and **B**).

Bony Cage (Fig. 17)

Clavicle should lay over third rib posteriorly. Costal cartilages are not seen unless calcified. The peculiarity of calcification of the costal cartilage is that in males, it makes a mottled appearance in the periphery and in females, it is central. Counting of ribs anteriorly and posteriorly should be practiced because they are important landmarks.

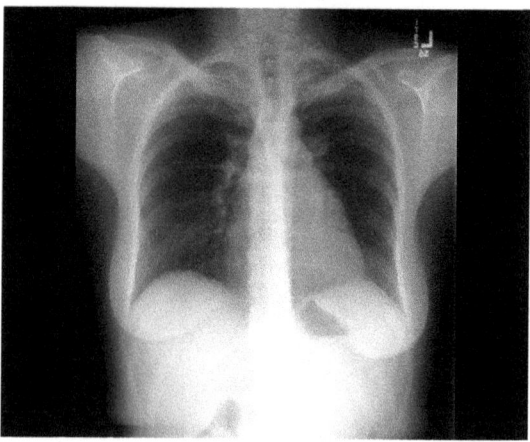

FIG. 11: Chest X-ray showing bilateral soft tissue (breast) shadows.

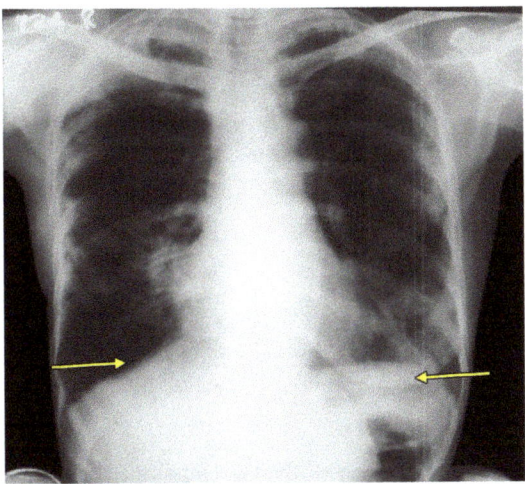

FIG. 12: Chest X-ray showing unilateral (right) absence of breast tissue shadow in a case of right mastectomy (yellow arrows).

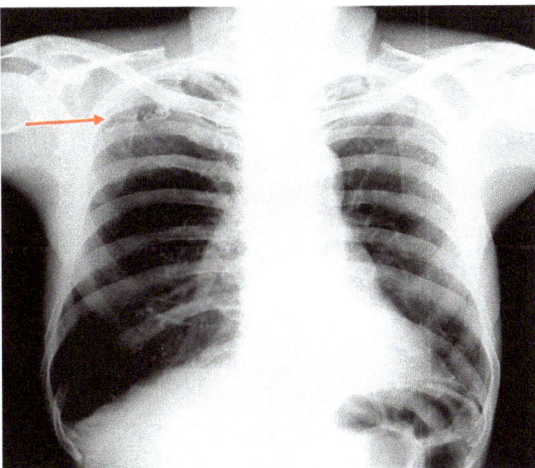

FIG. 13: Chest X-ray showing soft-tissue calcifications in the right side (parasitic infestation) (red arrow).

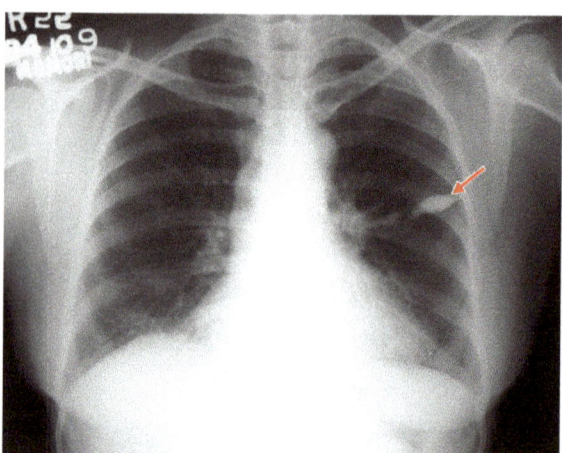

FIG. 14: Chest X-ray showing left chest wall subcutaneous calcifications (red arrow).

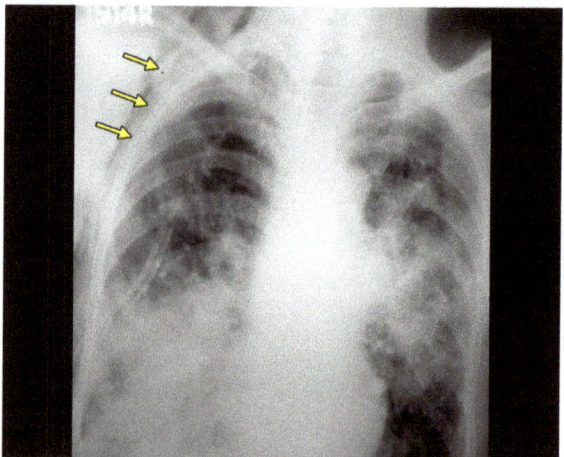

FIG. 15: Chest X-ray showing right chest wall subcutaneous emphysema with implantable cardioverter defibrillator (ICD) tube in situ (yellow arrows).

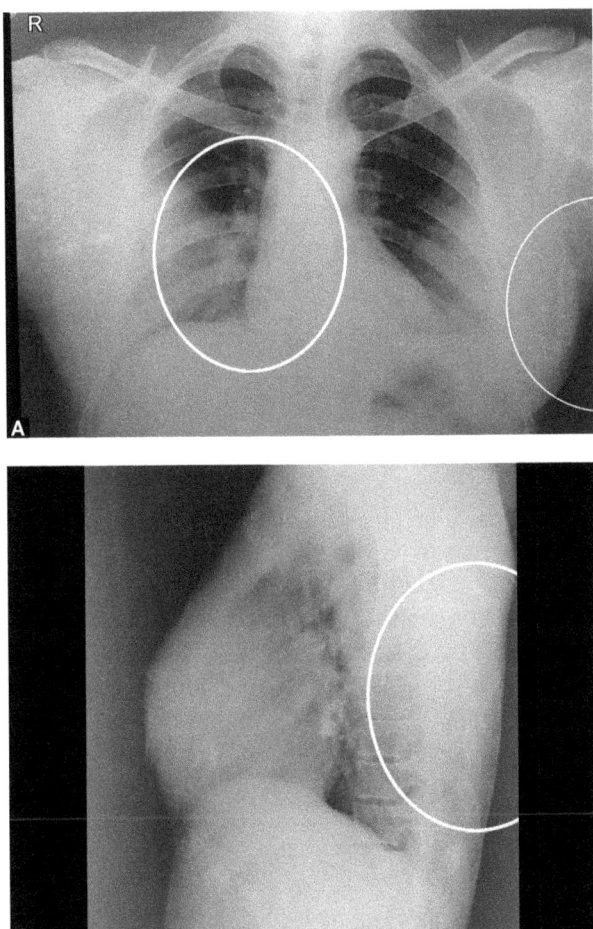

FIGS. 16A AND B: (A) Chest X-ray posteroanterior (PA) view showing soft-tissue density due to breast implant (silicon); and (B) Chest X-ray lateral view showing soft-tissue density due to breast implant (silicon).

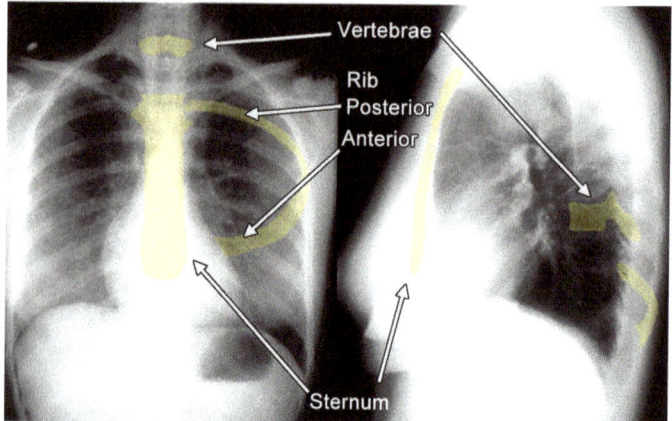

FIG. 17: Bony landmarks in normal chest X-ray.

Companion shadow is a faint soft-tissue shadow parallel to the clavicle or ribs resulting from overlying skin fold and subcutaneous tissue and has no pathological importance. Look for kyphoscoliosis, clavicular fracture, fracture of ribs, cervical ribs (**Fig. 18**), erosion of ribs, absent ribs, bifid ribs, fused ribs (**Fig. 19**), callous formation of ribs, and any bony mass (**Fig. 20**). Scapula is usually away from the lung field. Erosion of vertebra, absence of vertebra, fracture of vertebra, narrowing of disk space, and evidence of Pott's spine are also should be looked into.

Trachea and Mediastinum

Trachea appears as air-containing tube coming down from the sixth cervical vertebra and terminating at the carina where it bifurcates (T4-carina). The normal transverse internal diameter of the trachea ranges between 15 and 25 mm in men and 10 and 21 mm in women. On either sides of the trachea, the right and left paratracheal stripes are seen (**Fig. 21**).

Roentgenography: "A Step-by-step Approach to Reading of Chest X-ray" | 105

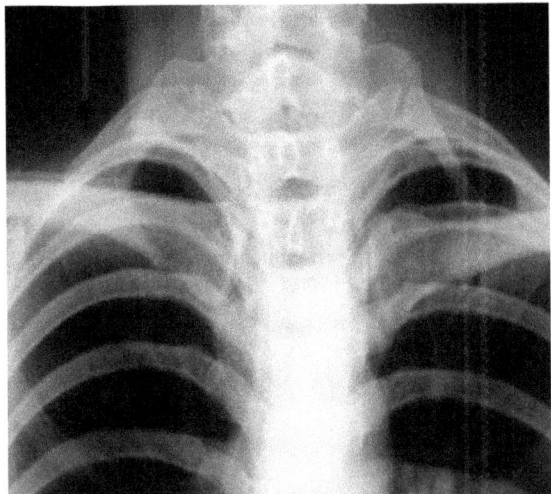

FIG. 18: Chest X-ray showing left cervical rib.

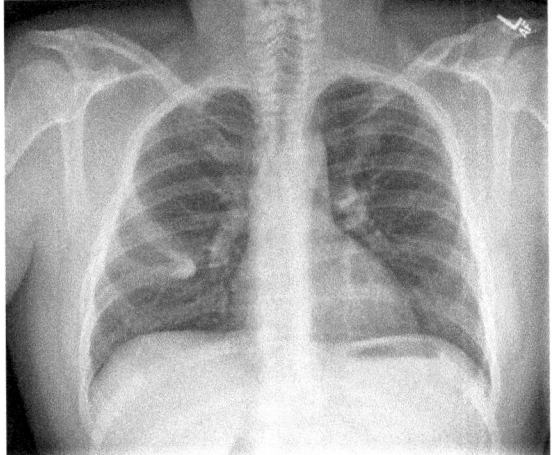

FIG. 19: Chest X-ray showing fusion of ribs (right fourth and fifth).

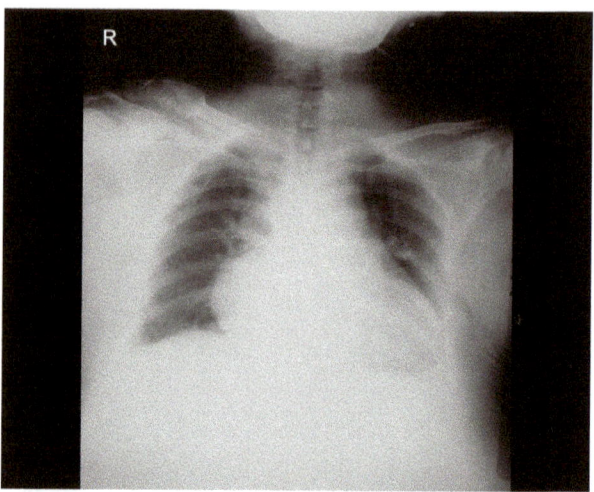

FIG. 20: Chest X-ray showing bony mass in the right clavicle.

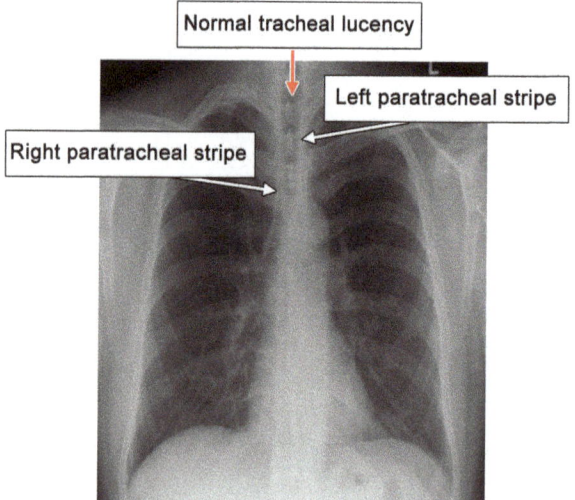

FIG. 21: Chest X-ray showing paratracheal stripes.

Abnormal thickening may be due to mediastinal pathology such as lymph node enlargement in lymphoma.

Tracheal position is usually central or with slight deviation to right that can be taken as normal provided no other pathology.

Reader has to look for retrosternal thyroid, paratracheal nodes, metastatic nodes, and rarely thymus.

Mediastinum

Superior Mediastinum or Upper Mediastinum

This is the part of mediastinum located above a horizontal line drawn from the angle of Louis to the spine posteriorly (**Fig. 22**). For reading the X-ray, the reader can consider upper mediastinum above the aortic knuckle.

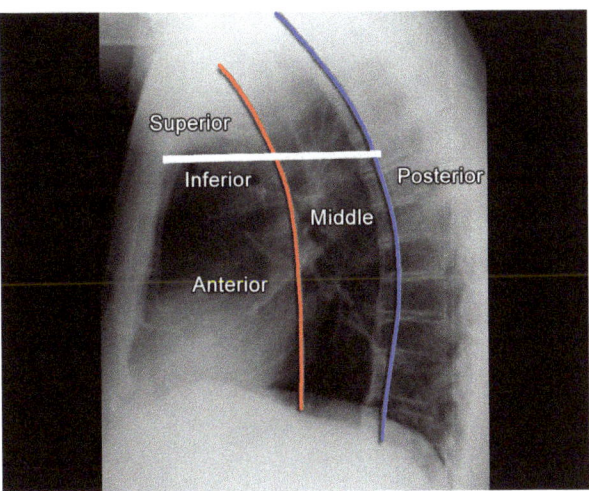

FIG. 22: Mediastinal compartments in chest X-ray.

Inferior/Lower Mediastinum

The compartments of inferior mediastinum with common diseases encountered in the mediastinum are depicted in **Figure 23**. An illustrative X-ray of a posterior mediastinal mass is shown in **Figures 24A** and **B**.

Heart

The right heart border is formed by the right atrium and the left heart border is formed by the left ventricle. The aortic

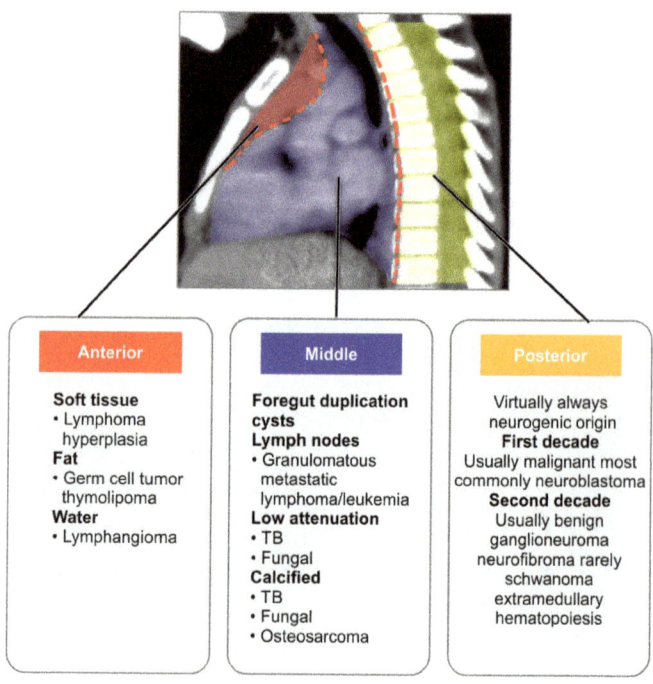

FIG. 23: Common diseases affecting the mediastinum.

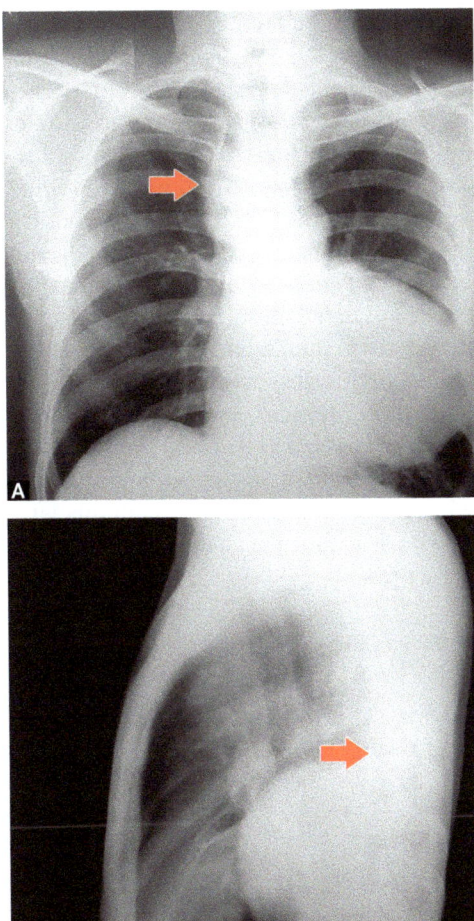

FIGS. 24A AND B: Chest radiograph appearance of posterior mediastinal mass in posteroanterior (PA) view (A) and lateral view (B). Arrow shows the right paratracheal node.

knuckle is an important anatomical landmark. The para-aortic line represents the left hand side of the descending thoracic aorta. It may be deviated in the elderly. Cardiac size is measured by drawing a line from the most lateral points of heart and another line drawn from the inner aspect of the widest points of the rib cage and the ratio is >50% that can be considered abnormal (**Fig. 25**). Cardiothoracic ratio ia approximately 15:33 cm and therefore within the normal limit of 50%. The normal cardiac size is approximately <15.5 cm in males and 14.5 cm in females. Increase in transverse cardiac diameter by 1.5 cm is significant. Cardiac shadow measuring >5.5 cm to the right signifies right atrial enlargement. The heart is said to be tubular if the maximum diameter is <11 cm on X-ray of the chest. Aortopulmonary window is the space located underneath the aortic arch (aortic knuckle) above the left pulmonary artery and contains fat. In the PA view, it appears as a concave shadow. It becomes convex, if adenopathy is present.

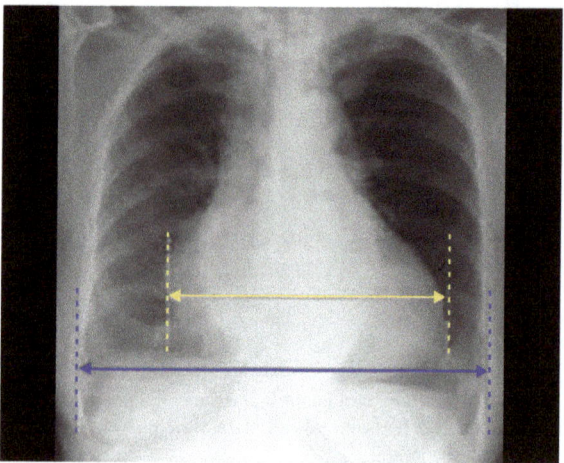

FIG. 25: Measurement of cardiac size in chest X-ray.

Causes of Increased Cardiothoracic Ratio

Obesity, pectus, portable film, cardiomegaly, and pericardial effusion.

Diaphragm

Diaphragm is dome-shaped and seen between 5th and 6th intercostal space. Right hemidiaphragm is 1.5–2 cm higher than the left hemidiaphragm. Costophrenic angles are acute and well-defined (**Fig. 26**). Any blunting of costophrenic angles may be due to pleural effusion (**Fig. 27**). Big breast also can cause obliteration because of the superimposed breast shadow. Cardiophrenic angle can be obliterated by pad of fat or any congenital cysts or mass.

Hilum

Chest X-ray assessment routinely involves checking the hilar structures for normal size, density, and position. The hila are

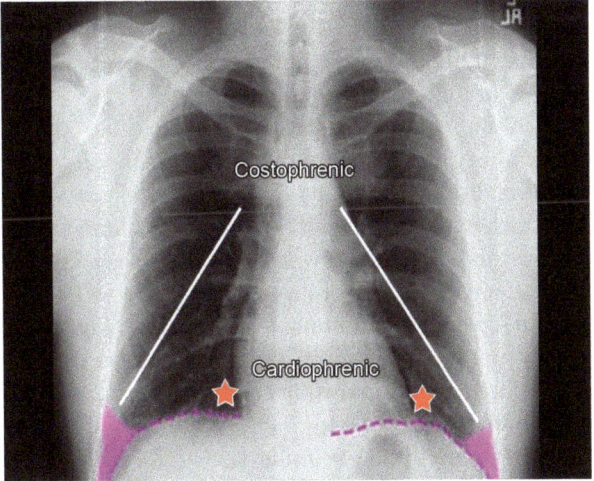

FIG. 26: Chest X-ray showing the costophrenic and cardiophrenic angles.

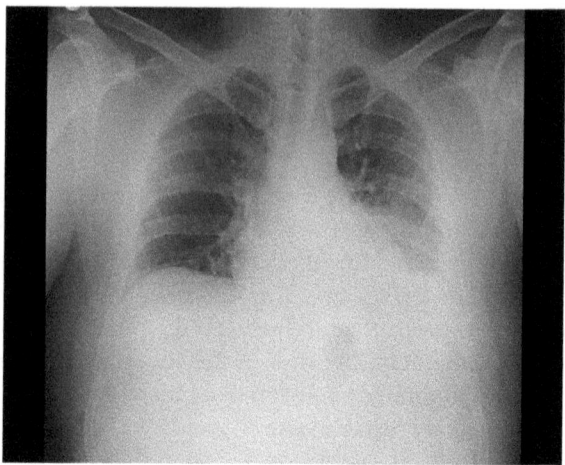

FIG. 27: Chest X-ray showing blunting of left costophrenic angle due to pleural effusion.

often wrongly called abnormal when normal and normal when abnormal. An awareness of the range of normal is important, but the best tip is to look for increase in density as well as size. If the hila are out of position, ask yourself if they are pushed or pulled or a rotated film.

The hilum contains anatomical structures containing the pulmonary vessels and the major bronchi, arranged asymmetrically and hilar lymph nodes are not normally visible. The left hilum is higher than the right hilum by 2.5 cm. Hilum—normal hilar shadow is made up of vessels and has concave shape. Each hilar point is the angle formed where the upper and lower lobe pulmonary vessels meet (**Fig. 28**). They are useful points of reference to determine the position of the hila. Not every normal subject has a clearly defined hilar point on both sides.

Both hila should be of similar size and density. If either hilum is bigger and more dense (whiter) than normal, this

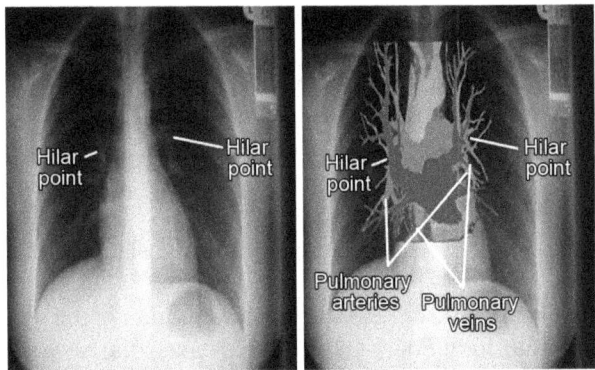

FIG. 28: Chest X-ray demonstrating the hilar points.

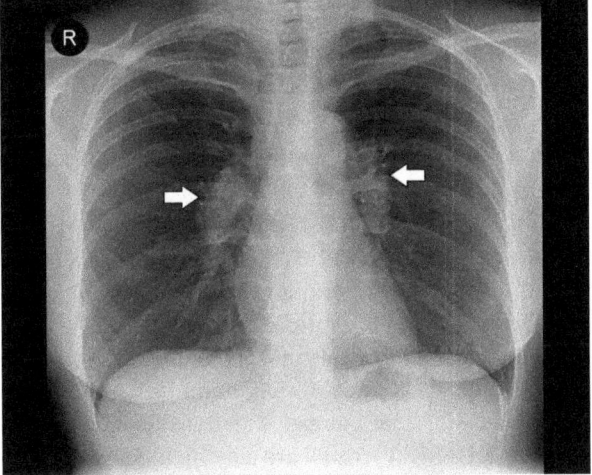

FIG. 29: Chest X-ray showing bilateral hilar enlargement due to adenopathy.

may indicate an abnormality (**Fig. 29**). The hilum is situated anteriorly at the level of the 3rd to 4th costal cartilage and posteriorly at the level of the T5–T7 vertebra.

One key difference between the hila is that:
- On the right, the right superior lobe bronchus divides from the right principal bronchus before the right hilum.
- On the left side, the left principal bronchus does not divide until it has entered the hilum of the lung.

Lung Fields

Divided into three zones for better anatomical localization of lesions.
1. Upper zone—from the apex to lower border of the second rib anteriorly (Why anteriorly? If taken the second rib posteriorly, there is no space—realize looking this at a PA view to convince yourself).
2. Mid zone—from the lower border of the second rib anteriorly to the lower border of the fourth rib anteriorly.
3. Lower zone—from the lower border of the fourth rib anteriorly to the level of diaphragm.

The fissures are mentioned below:
Horizontal fissure can be clearly seen in PA view. It extends from right hilum to the sixth rib in the axillary line. Oblique fissure is appreciated in the lateral view (right side). It starts from thoracic vertebra (T4–T5) to reach the diaphragm and 5 cm behind the costophrenic angle on the left and just behind the costophrenic angle on the right.

After localization of abnormal lesion in the lung, the next step is to identify the type of lesion. Commonly, abnormal lung lesions present either as increased air density or decreased air density (liquid density) which are classified below in **Table 2**.

Radiological Patterns of Lung Diseases
- Airspace opacity (**Fig. 30**)
- Interstitial opacity (**Fig. 31**)
- Nodules and masses (**Figs. 32** to **35**)

TABLE 2: Radiological patterns of lung diseases.

Decreased air density (liquid density)		Increased air density
Generalized	**Localized**	
• Diffuse alveolar	• Infiltrate	• Localized airway obstruction
• Diffuse interstitial	• Consolidation	• Diffuse airway obstruction
• Mixed	• Cavitation	• Emphysema
• Vascular	• Mass	• Bulla
	• Congestion	
	• Atelectasis/collapse	

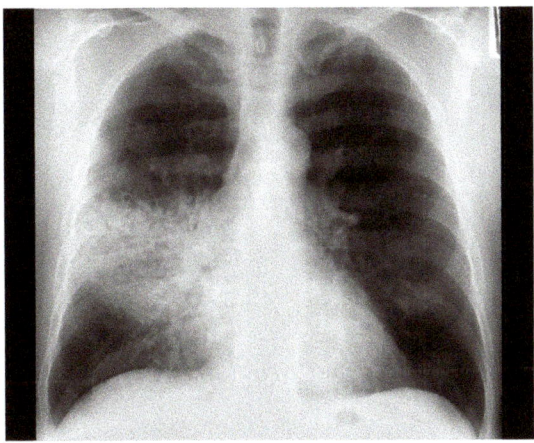

FIG. 30: Chest X-ray showing right middle and lower lobes airspace densities in a case of lower lobe pneumonia.

- Cysts and cavities (**Figs. 36** to **38**)
- Lung volumes (**Fig. 39**)
- Pleural diseases (**Fig. 40**)

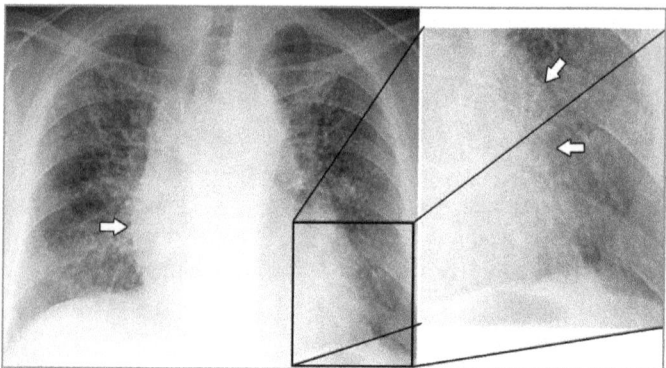

FIG. 31: Chest X-ray showing bilateral diffuse interstitial reticular densities in a case of interstitial lung disease.

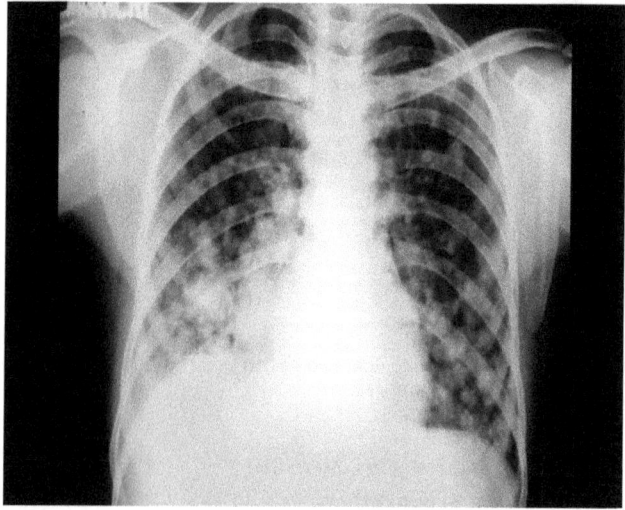

FIG. 32: Chest X-ray showing bilateral nodular densities in a case of lung secondaries.

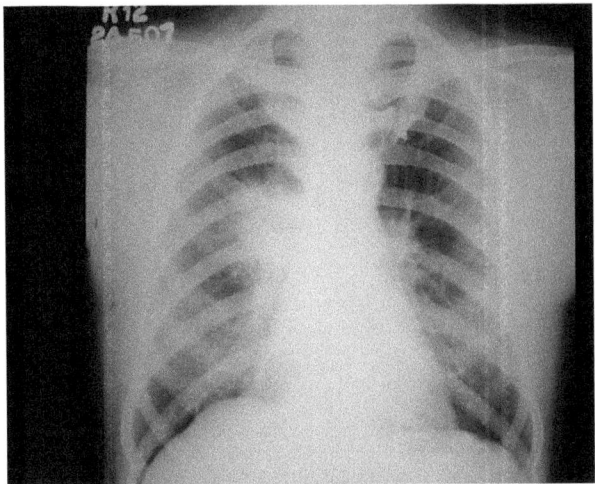

FIG. 33: Chest X-ray showing right lung mass lesion in a case of lung carcinoma.

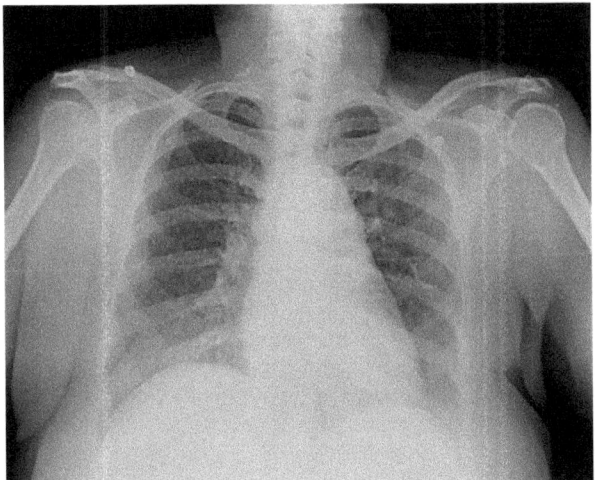

FIG. 34: Chest X-ray showing bilateral miliary shadows in disseminated tuberculosis in a patient with postmitral valve replacement surgery.

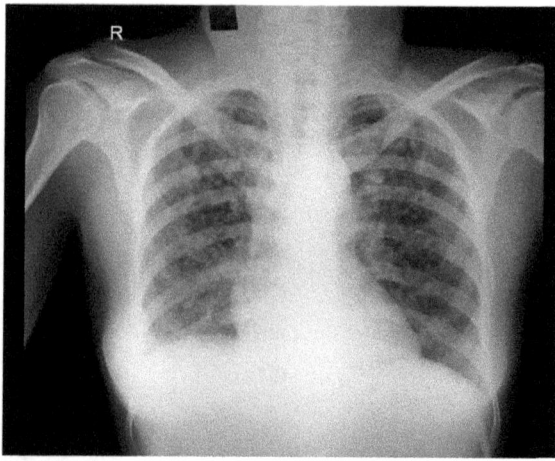

FIG. 34: Chest X-ray showing bilateral miliary shadows in disseminated tuberculosis in a patient with postmitral valve replacement surgery.

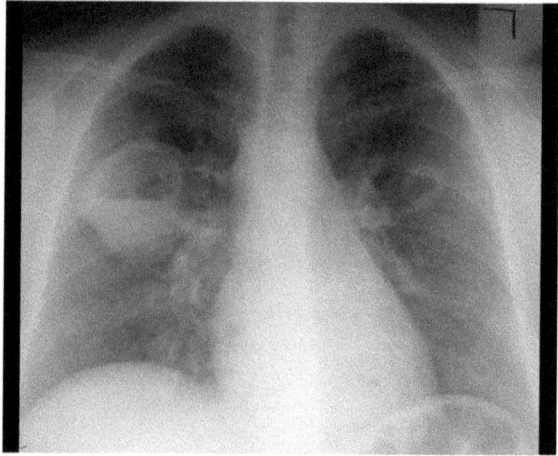

FIG. 35: Chest X-ray showing bilateral coarse miliary shadows in disseminated tuberculosis in a human immunodeficiency virus (HIV)-positive patient.

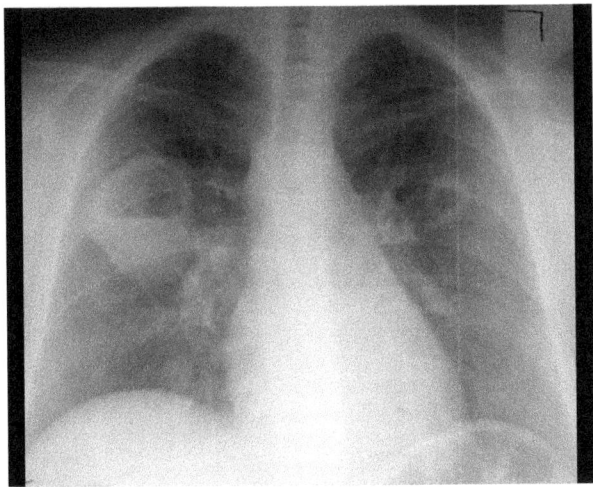

FIG. 36: Chest X-ray showing bilateral cavities in a case of pulmonary tuberculosis.

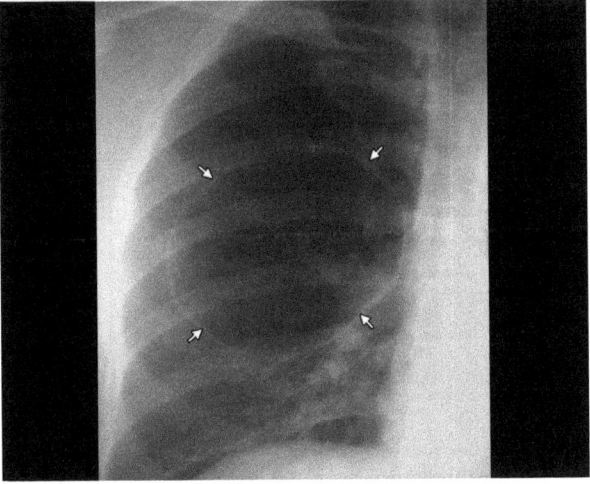

FIG. 37: Chest X-ray showing well-defined cystic lesion.

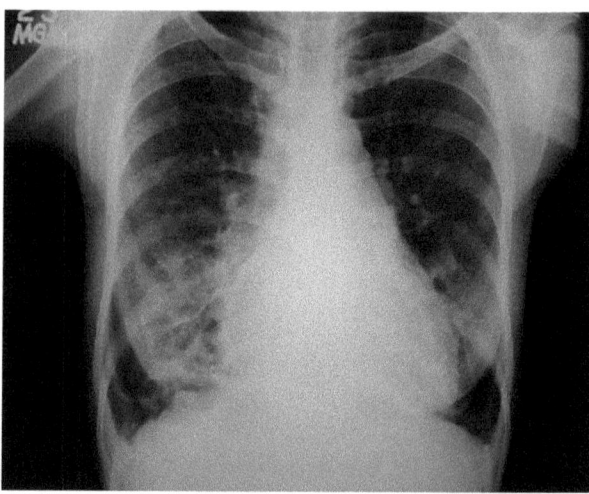

FIG. 38: Chest X-ray showing bilateral cystic lesions in a case of bronchiectasis.

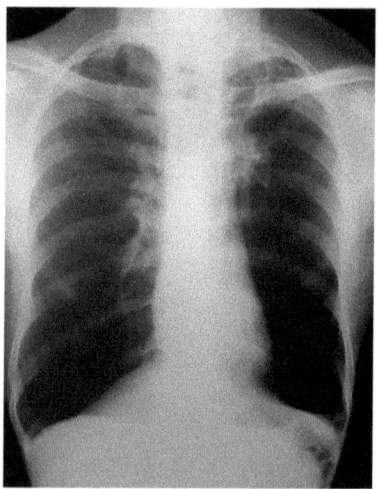

FIG. 39: Chest X-ray showing bilateral increase in lung volumes in a case of emphysema.

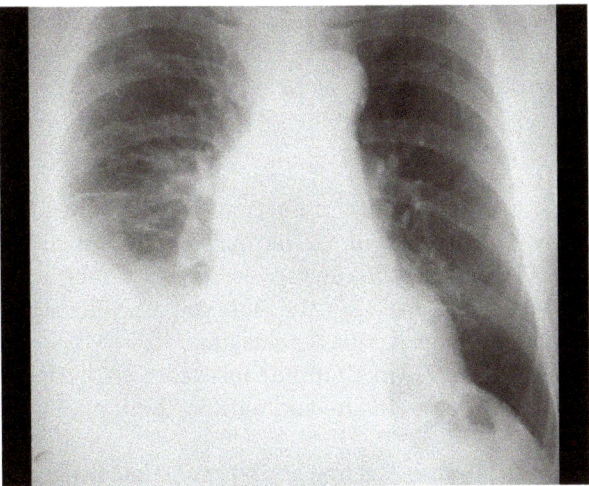

FIG. 40: Chest X-ray showing right pleural effusion.

Each of these patterns are nonspecific and can be presented by lung diseases of varying etiologies and pathologies. Also, there are classical radiological signs associated with these patterns for making differential diagnosis. The reader is advised to refer to radiology books for further reading.

PITFALLS OF CHEST X-RAY INTERPRETATION

- *Interpretation is technique dependent*:
  - Poor inspiratory film
  - Rotation
  - Over- or underpenetration
  - Error marking side
- *Inter-reader* variability occurs when X-ray readers disagree on the given X-ray where as *Intra-reader* variability occurs when a reader classifies a radiograph differently on different occasions. Reader variability is a draw back.

- *The hidden areas in the chest*: Lung apices, mediastinum, hila, and behind diaphragm cannot be completely evaluated using a CXR alone.

READING CHEST X-RAYS: TIPS

- The only way to learn to interpret CXRs is to read CXRs daily! Go through all the normal and abnormal X-rays published in this book and see more X-rays in the hospital. As we mentioned earlier, the more you see, you have more confidence interpreting the skiagram.
- Have a structured method! Be consistent with that method.
- Always check the name and date on the film (5% of the time it is wrong).
- Do not confuse "technical abnormalities" with pathological changes on a CXR.
- The CXR never lies!
- Ask for help in case of doubt in interpreting X-ray, it is always available!
- The obvious is not always the most important finding! Also, never look at the X-ray >2 minutes—otherwise you see many things which are not there.
- And keep the customary 6 feet while reading the X-ray!

Keep the safe distance.

CHAPTER 6

Management of Pulmonary Emergencies

ACUTE EXACERBATION OF BRONCHIAL ASTHMA

In a well-controlled asthmatic on medication, a sudden deterioration with increased breathlessness, the patient is advised to consult the nearest doctor or hospital. Infections and exposure to allergens are the most important cause of exacerbation. Pneumothorax should always be considered as one of the important factors for increased dyspnea.

Investigations

- Peak expiratory flow rate (PEFR)
- Forced expiratory volume in one second (FEV1) (if the patient can do it)—if the accessory muscles of respiration is in action, it indicates 30% reduction in FEV1.
- Oxygen saturation (SpO_2)
- Arterial blood gas (ABG)

Moderate Exacerbation of Asthma

Any one of the criteria:
- Increasing symptoms.
- Peak expiratory flow >50–75% best or predicted or <200 L/min.

- Wheezing heard on auscultation.
- No features of acute severe asthma.

Acute Severe Asthma

Any one of the criteria:
- Peak expiratory flow 33–50% best or predicted or <80 L/min.
- Respiratory rate ≥25 breaths/min.
- Heart rate ≥110 beats/min.
- Use of accessory muscles.
- Inability to complete sentences in one breath.
- Wheezing heard on auscultation.

Life-threatening Asthma

Any one of the criteria:
- Peak expiratory flow <33% best or predicted.
- Oxygen saturation <92%.
- Partial pressure of arterial oxygen (PaO_2) <60 mm Hg on oxygen.
- Partial pressure of arterial carbon dioxide ($PaCO_2$) >45 mm Hg on oxygen.
- Silent chest (no wheezes heard because of severe bronchospasm).
- Pulsus paradoxus >15 mm Hg.
- Look for pneumothorax.
- Cyanosis
- Poor respiratory effort.
- Arrhythmia
- Exhaustion and altered conscious level.

Near-fatal Asthma

- Raised $PaCO_2$ and/or requiring mechanical ventilation with raised inflation pressures.

Criteria for Admission

- Admit patients with any feature of a life-threatening or near-fatal attack.
- Admit patients with any feature of a severe attack persisting after initial treatment.
- Normal or increased $PaCO_2$ or a decreased pH implies potentially life-threatening situation.
- Partial pressure of arterial oxygen <50 mm Hg.
- Radiological evidence of pneumothorax and consolidation.
- Patients whose peak flow is >75% best or predicted 1 hour after initial treatment may be discharged from casualty, unless there are other reasons which require admission.

Clinical Features

Severe breathlessness (including too breathless to complete sentences in one breath), tachypnea, tachycardia, wheeze or silent chest (due to acute bronchospasm), cyanosis, or collapse.

None of these singly or together is specific and their absence does not exclude a severe attack.

Investigations

Peak Expiratory Flow or Forced Expiratory Volume in One Second

Peak expiratory flow or FEV1 is useful and valid measures of airway caliber.

Pulse Oximetry

Oxygen saturation measured by pulse oximetry determines the adequacy of oxygen therapy and the need for ABG. The aim of oxygen therapy is to maintain SpO_2 94–98%.

Blood Gases (Arterial Blood Gas)

Patients with SpO_2 <92% or other features of life-threatening asthma require ABG measurement.

Chest X-ray

Chest X-ray (CXR) is recommended:
- Suspected pneumomediastinum or pneumothorax
- Suspected consolidation
- Life-threatening asthma
- Failure to respond to treatment satisfactorily.
- Requirement for ventilation.

Treatment

Oxygen
- Give supplementary oxygen to all hypoxemic patients with acute asthma to maintain an SpO_2 level of 94–98%.
- Lack of pulse oximetry should not prevent the use of oxygen.
- In hospital, ambulance, and primary care, nebulized β2-agonist bronchodilators should be driven by oxygen.
- The absence of supplemental oxygen should not prevent nebulized therapy being given, if indicated.

β2-agonist

Use high-dose inhaled β2-agonists as first-line agents in acute asthma and administer as early as possible. Reserve intravenous (IV) β2-agonists (more tachycardia) for those patients in whom inhaled therapy cannot be used reliably.
- In patients with severe asthma—that is poorly responsive to an initial bolus dose of β2-agonist, consider continuous nebulization with an appropriate nebulizer.

- In acute asthma with life-threatening features, the nebulized route (oxygen driven) is recommended.

Steroid Therapy
- Inhaled steroids.
- Intravenous methylprednisolone 1 mg/kg or 40 mg 6th hourly/hydrocortisone hemisuccinate 200 mg stat followed by 100 mg 6th hourly.
- Give steroids in adequate doses in all cases of acute asthma. Continue prednisolone 40–50 mg daily for at least 5 days or until recovery.

Ipratropium Bromide
Add nebulized ipratropium bromide (0.5 mg stat and 6th to 8th hourly). Add to β2-agonist treatment for patients with acute severe or life-threatening asthma or those with a poor to initial response to β2-agonist therapy [but more useful in chronic obstructive pulmonary disease (COPD)].

Other Therapies
- Intravenous methylxanthines—aminophylline (as bolus dosage or drip—blood levels to be kept between 10 and 15 µg/mL) or IV deriphyllin.
- Consider giving a single dose of IV magnesium sulfate for patients with acute severe asthma who have not had a good initial response to inhaled bronchodilator therapy, life-threatening or near-fatal asthma with FEV1 of 25–30%.

Intravenous magnesium sulfate (2 g in 100 mL normal saline IV infusion over 20 min) should only be used with caution.
- Routine prescription of antibiotics is not indicated for patients with acute asthma.

- Heliox
- Intravenous leukotriene antagonists
- Correct dehydration
- No sedation.
- Inhaled mucolytics are not advised in severe cases as they may worsen cough.

Good Response

- Sustained response after 60 minutes.
- Physical examination near normal and patient having no distress.
- Peak expiratory flow >70%.
- Oxygen saturation >95%.

After observing the patient for few hours, he/she can be discharged with the advice to continue with metered-dose inhaler containing inhaled corticosteroids and long-acting β2-agonist.

Oral steroids are to be continued for 7–10 days is ideal tapering over days.

If patient is not responding to the aggressive therapy after 6–12 hours, refer to intensive care.

Refer any patient:
- Requiring ventilatory support.
- *With acute, severe, or life-threatening asthma, failing to respond to therapy, evidenced by*:
  - Deteriorating PEF (<30%).
  - Persisting or worsening hypoxia
  - Hypercapnia
  - Arterial blood gas analysis showing decreased pH.
  - Exhaustion and feeble respiration
  - Drowsiness, confusion, and altered conscious state.
  - Respiratory arrest

Intubation

Exhausted patient with increase in $PaCO_2$ and developing progressive respiratory acidosis. Initial PaO_2 over 50 mm Hg and pH around 7.30 and if the patient is alert and cooperative may not require intubation.

If the patient requires ventilatory support:

- Mode can be either assist control or synchronized intermittent mandatory ventilation (SIMV).
- Tidal volume given should be 5–8 mL/kg.
- Initial rate should be 6–10 breaths/min.
- Peak inspiratory flow rate should be 70–90 L/min.
- End-inspiratory plateau pressure to be kept below 35 cm of H_2O.
- Positive end-expiratory pressure (PEEP) adjusted to 75–80% of measured auto-PEEP level.
- Fraction of inspired oxygen (FiO_2) to be kept to maintain $PaCO_2$.
- Sedation to prevent tachypnea and allows the patient to rest during the first 24 hours.

Permissive hypercapnia protects the lung from ventilator-induced lung injury by using smaller than usual tidal volumes and limiting alveolar distending pressure. β2-agonist therapy to be continued during mechanical ventilation with higher doses because of the deposition of drug on the walls of endotracheal tube.

Complications expected are—barotrauma, prolonged muscle weakness due to high doses of steroids, and muscle relaxants.

The patient is discharged with the advice to continue with metered-dose inhaler containing inhaled corticosteroids and long-acting β2-agonist.

Oral steroids are to be continued for 7–10 days.

Patient should be advised to use peak flow meter in the morning and evening and if there is a fall advised to approach the treating physician.

Nebulizer Solutions Available

- *Salbutamol:* 1 mL of salbutamol solution contains 5 mg of salbutamol.
- *Budesonide:* 2 mL solution contains 0.5 mg.
- *Ipratropium bromide:* 250 µg/mL.
- *Fluticasone:* 0.5 mg in 2 mL.
- Combination of formoterol 0.5 mg and budesonide 1 mg in 2 mL.
- Combination of ipratropium bromide (500 µg) and levosalbutamol (1.25 mg) in 2.5 mL.

In ultrasonic nebulizers, only solution can be delivered and not suspension (budesonide is available in suspension form).

ACUTE EXACERBATION OF CHRONIC OBSTRUCTIVE PULMONARY DISEASE

In a COPD patient, the precipitating factors can be infections, weather changes, nonadherence to medications, inhalation of tobacco smoke, air pollution, etc.

Sudden onset of symptoms such as:
- Increase in cough.
- Increase in breathlessness.
- Increase in sputum volume and change in its color (white to green, yellow, or blood-streaked).
- Fever
- Chest pain

- Increased tiredness.
- Increase in oxygen requirement (for those on long-term oxygen therapy).
- Altered sensorium.

Usually, patients present with varying combination of these symptoms. During clinical assessment, objective evaluation is necessary to assess severity of underlying COPD, the presence of comorbidities, and history of previous exacerbation. The physical examination should evaluate the effect of the episode on hemodynamic and respiratory systems.

Investigations

Look for the following:
- Use of accessory muscles
- Paradoxical chest movements
- Central cyanosis
- Systolic pressure <90 mm Hg
- Respiratory rate 30 breaths/min or more
- Heart rate >110 beats/min
- Altered mental status
- Asterixis (flapping tremor)
- Severe comorbid conditions
- Oxygen saturation <90%

Exclude:
- Pneumonia
- Pneumothorax
- Pulmonary embolism
- Paroxysmal atrial tachycardia (arrhythmias)
- Pulmonary edema
- Pleural effusion
- Associated cor pulmonale

Presence of any one of the abovementioned signs is an indicator for hospital admission.

The diagnostic procedures to perform such as chest radiology, sputum and blood examination, ABG, and serum electrolytes. Spirometry may not be possible.

Treatment to Follow

- Bronchodilators
- Steroids
- Antibiotics
- Oxygen therapy
- Mechanical ventilation—noninvasive or invasive

TENSION PNEUMOTHORAX

A tension pneumothorax is a complete collapse of the lung. It occurs when air enters, but does not leave the pleural space.

Causes

Any condition that leads to pneumothorax can cause a tension pneumothorax. In uncomplicated pneumothorax, air can enter and leave the pleural space easily. In tension pneumothorax, however, air enters the pleural space with each breath and gets trapped there.

As the amount of trapped air increases, pressure builds up in the chest. The lung collapses on that side and can push the important structures in the center of the chest (such as the heart, major blood vessels, and airways) toward the other side of the chest. The shift can cause the other lung to become compressed and can affect the flow of blood returning to the heart and the lung excursion of the opposite side also is compromised.

This situation can lead to low blood pressure, shock, and death.

Symptoms
- Sudden chest pain
- Dyspnea
- Chest tightness
- Cyanosis
- Tachycardia
- Hypotension
- Decreased mental alertness
- Tachypnea
- Bulging (distended) veins in the neck
- Profuse sweating

Examination

Patient in distress with the above symptoms as it is a medical emergency. If suspected, percussion (hyperresonant note) and on auscultation the breath sounds are decreased. Mediastinal shift may be noted. There may be subcutaneous emphysema.

Tests used to diagnose tension pneumothorax include:
- Chest X-ray
- Arterial blood gases
- Electrocardiogram

Treatment

Treatment is aimed to remove the air from the pleural space, allowing the lung to re-expand. In an emergency, a small needle (such as a standard IV needle) may be placed into the chest cavity through the ribs to relieve pressure.

The standard treatment is an intercostal tube with water seal. The chest tube is attached to a vacuum bottle that slowly removes air from the chest cavity. This allows the lung to re-expand. As the lung heals and stops leaking air, the vacuum is turned down and then the chest tube is removed. Sometimes, it can take several days for the affected lung to fully re-expand.

Pleurodesis—if the problem happens again or if the lung does not re-expand after 5 days with a chest tube in place.

Prognosis

Up to 50% of patients who had pneumothorax may have recurrence. There are no long-term complications after a successful treatment.

Possible Complications

- Acute respiratory failure
- Air in the mediastinal space, which can interfere with heart and lung function (pneumomediastinum).
- Very low blood pressure (shock).
- Death

HEMOPTYSIS

Hemoptysis is coughing of blood.

Identify Which Side is Bleeding

By past history of respiratory illness and treatment usually volunteered by the patient and by auscultation (e.g., post-tubercular right upper lobe bronchiectasis)—presence of crackles, old X-rays.

Quantification is given in the earlier chapter.

Position

Patient whose right lung is bleeding should be placed in the right side down decubitus position (with head end low) whereas a patient whose left lung is bleeding should be placed in the left side down decubitus position (with head end low). The purpose of these positions is to protect the nonbleeding lung, since spillage of blood into the nonbleeding lung may prevent gas exchange by blocking the airway with clot or filling the alveoli with blood.

Guidelines for the Management of Hemoptysis

Initial Management
- *Airway*: Establishing patent airway by intubation.
- Breathing
- *Circulation:* If the patient cannot maintain his/her airway—intubation.
- Make the patient lie on the same side as lesion/abnormality on CXR.
- Intravenous access and volume replacement.
- Hemostatic (controversial role)
- Blood for cross-match, complete blood count, and clotting time.
- *Hemoptysis:* >150 mL airway compromise.

Further Assessment
- Bronchoscopy
- CT thorax for anatomical localization.

Management
- Bronchial arterial embolization/surgery/bronchoscopy (rigid or flexible) to identify source of bleeding.
- Assume infection in patients with cystic fibrosis/bronchiectasis and treat aggressively with antibiotics.

RESPIRATORY FAILURE

All patients require ABG, ECG, and X-ray of chest.

Respiratory failure occurs when pulmonary gas exchange is impaired resulting in hypoxemia (PaO_2 <60 mm Hg) with or without hypercarbia ($PaCO_2$ >55 mm Hg).

Classification

- Type I or hypoxemic respiratory failure.
- Type II or hypercapnic respiratory failure.
- Type III or perioperative respiratory failure.
- Type IV or respiratory failure associated with shock.

Type I Respiratory Failure

- Characterized by an arterial oxygen tension (PaO_2) lower than 60 mm Hg with a normal or low arterial carbon dioxide tension ($PaCO_2$).
- This is the most common form of respiratory failure.
- There are two mechanisms described in the pathophysiology:
  i. Ventilation-perfusion mismatch
  ii. Right-to-left shunt
- The common clinical features include sweating, restlessness, anxiety, tachycardia, and tachypnea.
- This is seen in various conditions such as pneumonia, pulmonary edema, pneumothorax, and pulmonary emboli.

Management

- Maintain a patent airway.
- Supplementary oxygenation
- Principles of ventilatory support—administration of PEEP.

- Identification and treatment of the primary condition (for further details, refer prescribed textbooks).

Type II Respiratory Failure

- Also called ventilatory respiratory failure or pump failure.
- It is characterized by a $PaCO_2$ higher than 55 mm Hg.
- Hypoxemia is also common in patients with hypercapnic respiratory failure.
- The mechanism of pathophysiology is alveolar hypoventilation.

This may be due to:
- Reduced ventilatory effort.
- Inability to overcome an increased resistance to ventilation.
- Failure to compensate for increase in dead space or increased carbon dioxide production.

The common clinical features include sweating, bounding pulse, tachycardia, headache, flapping tremors, and drowsiness.

It can be further classified into:
- Acute
- Acute on chronic
- Chronic

Acute: It refers to an acute rise in $PaCO_2$ level, a rise in H^+ level, and a fall in pH level.

Acute on chronic: There is a fall in pH level due to acutely increased $PaCO_2$ level associated with chronic elevated HCO_3^- levels.

Chronic: Normal pH levels are associated with chronically elevated $PaCO_2$ and HCO_3^- levels.

- Acute and acute on chronic types are seen in acute exacerbations of COPD.

- Chronic type is seen in conditions such as COPD, obesity hypoventilation syndrome, and motor neuron disease.

Management
- Maintain a patent airway.
- Principles of ventilatory support—administration of pressure support.
- Identification and treatment of the primary condition (for further details, refer prescribed textbooks).

Type III Respiratory Failure
- Occurs as a result of lung atelectasis and is seen commonly in the perioperative period.
- After general anesthesia, decrease in functional residual capacity leads to collapse of dependent lung units and subsequent hypoventilation.

Management
- Frequent change in position.
- Chest physiotherapy
- Adequate analgesia
- Principles of ventilatory support—administration of PEEP to reverse regional atelectasis.

Type IV Respiratory Failure
- Occurs due to hypoperfusion of respiratory muscles in patients with shock.
- Patients in shock suffer respiratory distress because of hypoperfusion resulting in lactic acidosis.

Management
- Correction of shock.
- Invasive mechanical ventilation (noninvasive ventilation is contraindicated as PEEP may worsen the hypotension).

CHAPTER 7

Viva Voce Questions and Bedside Questions

INTRODUCTION

Approaching the stage of life when you would be appearing in front of external examiners for the first time? Sure no! From 1st year of medical education, they sit opposite with a sneer. Feeling the fright of answering several questions and explaining? If you are getting cold feet, then do not worry. You do not need to exhaust yourself pondering over what the viva questions would be like and how you would establish your credentials in the examinations because we are here with some of the popularly asked questions that you must be prepared for.

VIVA VOCE QUESTIONS

1. Indications for bronchoscopy before lung resection.
2. Continuous diaphragm sign.
3. Change in voice in inhaled corticosteroids (ICS) usage.
4. Indications of clarithromycin.
5. Ranke's complex.
6. Clinical importance of lymphatic drainage of left lower lobe.

7. Adverse effects of isoniazid.
8. Eggshell calcification.
9. Side effects of fluoroquinolones.
10. Monday morning fever.
11. Spirometric patterns in acute hypersensitivity pneumonitis (HP).
12. Teardrop sign.
13. White-out lung.
14. Cole's vicious cycle hypothesis.
15. What is air quality index?
16. Causes of bilateral diaphragmatic paralysis.
17. Conditions associated with Hamman's crunch.
18. Reverse halo sign.
19. Casoni's test.
20. Falling lung sign.
21. Why sunlight should be avoided in sarcoidosis?
22. Erythema nodosum.
23. Radiological demonstration of small pneumothorax.
24. Biot's breathing.
25. Which antitubercular drug inhibits theophylline metabolism?
26. Bulging fissure sign.
27. Deep sulcus.
28. Most frequent paraneoplastic syndrome associated with small cell lung cancer.
29. Lambert–Eaton myasthenic syndrome.
30. At what age, the fall in forced expiratory volume in one second (FEV1) starts?
31. Where will you see primary complex in congenital tuberculosis?
32. Average rate of lung expansion in pneumothorax physiologically.

33. Complications of bronchiectasis.
34. Indications of rifampicin.
35. Side effects of ethionamide.
36. What is "fall and rise" phenomenon?
37. Alternative to Mantoux test.
38. Yellow nail syndrome.
39. Types of pulmonary edema and radiological differences.
40. Vanishing lung syndrome.
41. Troisier's sign.
42. Autologous blood transfusion.
43. Re-expansion pulmonary edema.
44. Caplan's syndrome.
45. Oxygen toxicity.
46. Cholesterol pleural effusion.
47. Cobb angle.
48. Salvage therapy.
49. Side effects of steroids.
50. Acute cor pulmonale.
51. Luftsichel sign.
52. Reverse Robin Hood effect.
53. Heliox.
54. Wasted perfusion.
55. Differential diagnosis of asthma.
56. Types of emphysema.
57. Antigenic shift and drift.
58. Comorbidities of chronic obstructive pulmonary disease (COPD).
59. Normal serum levels of theophylline.
60. Stages of allergic bronchopulmonary aspergillosis (ABPA).
61. Contraindications of pleural tap.
62. Cepacia syndrome.
63. Differential diagnosis of miliary mottling.

64. Conditions associated with smoking-related interstitial lung disease (SR-ILD).
65. Apnea-hypopnea index.
66. Radiological signs of pulmonary embolism.
67. What are the three types of disordered breathing?
68. Golden "S" sign.
69. Tests for primary ciliary dyskinesia.
70. Sterilizing drugs in tuberculosis (TB).
71. Why there is poor response to inhaled corticosteroids (ICS) in smokers?
72. Pseudochylothorax.
73. Steroids in tuberculosis (TB).
74. Hamman–Rich syndrome.
75. Bedside tests for pulmonary function.
76. Water lily appearance.
77. Causes of unilateral elevation of diaphragm.
78. Trapped lung.
79. Smoking cessation.
80. Walking pneumonia.
81. Exercise-induced bronchoconstriction.
82. Define cavity and importance of cavity wall thickness.
83. Stages of sarcoidosis.
84. Nonpulmonary causes of cor pulmonale.
85. Causes of pyothorax turning to pyopneumothorax.
86. Sites of encysted pleural effusion.
87. Differential diagnosis of lung abscess.
88. Oxygen toxicity.
89. Rosenberg–Patterson classification.
90. Sail sign.
91. Unresolved pneumonia.
92. Unilateral hyperlucency in X-ray.
93. Morgagni's hernia.

94. Lamellar effusion.
95. CT angiogram sign.
96. Vanishing lung syndrome.
97. Re-expansion pulmonary edema (complications of paracentesis thoracis).
98. Kinyoun stain
99. Paraneoplastic syndrome associated with small cell carcinoma.
100. Comorbidities of sleep disordered breathing.
101. Lübeck disaster.
102. Antigravity aspiration.
103. Vaccines in chronic obstructive pulmonary disease (COPD).
104. Stains used for diagnosing *Pneumocystis jiroveci* pneumonia (PJP).
105. Accessory muscles of respiration.
106. Platypnea.
107. Bucket handle and pump handle.
108. Advantage of pursed lip breathing.
109. Drugs causing gynecomastia.
110. Ortner's syndrome.
111. Poland's syndrome.
112. Cannon ball shadows.
113. Bilateral hilar enlargement.
114. Unresolved pneumonia.
115. Kerley lines.
116. Hoover's sign.
117. Cervicothoracic sign.
118. Pirfenidone.
119. Samter's triad.
120. Primary lung abscess.
121. Glycopyrronium.

122. Bronchoalveolar lavage.
123. Pleurodesis.
124. Camelot's sign.
125. Drug-induced psychosis.
126. Iloprost.
127. Atoll sign.
128. Pneumatocele.
129. Different types of nebulizers.
130. Complications of pneumonia.
131. Radiation pneumonitis.
132. Management of hemoptysis.
133. Causes of chronic empyema.
134. Tietze syndrome.
135. Pseudochylothorax.
136. Reverse halo sign.
137. Phantom tumor.
138. Ipsilateral pulmonary edema.
139. Assessment of weaning a patient from ventilator.
140. Contralateral pulmonary edema.
141. Young's syndrome.
142. Complications of asthma.
143. Home oxygen therapy.
144. Causes of spontaneous pneumothorax.
145. Differential diagnosis of solitary pulmonary nodule (SPN)—at least five causes.
146. Contraindication of radiotherapy in bronchus cancer.
147. Dressler's syndrome.
148. Meigs and Pseudo-Meigs syndrome.
149. Causes of honeycomb lung.
150. Clinical effects of mediastinal tumor.
151. Cold abscess.
152. Measuring height in kyphoscoliosis.

153. Causes of diaphragmatic paralysis.
154. Sniff test.
155. Wells score.
156. Aclidinium.
157. What are the screening guidelines for chronic obstructive pulmonary disease (COPD)?
158. Mendelson's syndrome.
159. Orthodeoxia.

CLINICAL EXAMINATION QUESTIONS

1. Signs of protein-energy malnutrition (PEM).
2. Clinical signs of hair in kwashiorkor and marasmus.
3. Vitamins and deficiencies.
4. External markers of tuberculosis (TB).
5. Ocular manifestations of tuberculosis (TB).
6. Midarm circumference (MAC) range.
7. Obesity classification.
8. Objective criteria for built and nourishment.
9. Upper airway definition.
10. Mallampati and Modified Mallampati classification.
11. Importance of uvula in obstructive sleep apnea (OSA).
12. Why to examine ear in RS (clinical significance)?
13. Impacted wax in ear (clinical significance).
14. Causes of chronic cough.
15. Why tobacco stains is predisposed to canine teeth?
16. Recurrent uvular edema—causes.
17. Causes of superior vena cava (SVC) syndrome.
18. Other name for apical impulse.
19. How to make apical impulse visualized/felt?
20. Jugular venous pressure (JVP).
21. Pulsatile and nonpulsatile jugular venous pressure (JVP).

22. Digital index.
23. Respiratory causes of pedal edema.
24. Common sites of tuberculosis (TB).
25. How bronchogenic carcinoma gets to scalene node?
26. Clinical triad of tuberculosis (TB) lymph nodes.
27. Jones and Campbell classification.
28. Apical impulse in right ventricular hypertrophy (RVH), left ventricular hypertrophy (LVH), and cor pulmonale.
29. Abnormalities of sternum.
30. Abnormalities of angle of Louis.
31. Anatomical significance in angle of Louis.
32. Why is pectus excavatum more detrimental?
33. Flail chest.
34. Tietze syndrome.
35. What is tracheal descent/tracheal tug?
36. Mechanism of tracheal tug.
37. Subcostal angle.
38. How to measure chest expansion?
39. Causes of chest wall tenderness.
40. Nerve supply of pleura.
41. Anatomy of lung and pleura.
42. Adams-Oliver syndrome.
43. What are turbulent and laminar flow and hertz in each?
44. Palpable rales.
45. Superior vena cava (SVC) obstruction.
46. Thoracic duct—course, level of injury, and interpretation.
47. Anatomical significance at T4.
48. Lines of the chest.
49. Midpoint of clavicle and midclavicular point.
50. Tidal percussion versus liver dullness.
51. Surrogate marker of PP ratio.
52. Other causes of pallor.

53. Respiratory conditions associated with icterus.
54. Differences between central and peripheral cyanosis.
55. Mixed cyanosis.
56. Mechanism of cyanosis.
57. Mechanism of clubbing.
58. Percentage of bronchiectasis patients with clubbing.
59. Definition of paraneoplastic syndrome.
60. Conditions in which clubbing is seen in tuberculosis (TB).
61. Waveforms in jugular venous pressure (JVP).
62. Vitamin deficiency and external markers.
63. Bitot's spots and phlycten.
64. Angular cheilitis and stomatitis.
65. Vitamin D and respiratory system examination.
66. Fall by crisis and fall by lysis.
67. Causes of evening rise of temperature.
68. Fever and hyperthermia.
69. Fever types.
70. Infrared thermometer—mechanism.
71. Interpretation of infrared thermometer readings.
72. How will you elicit character of pulse?
73. Bradycardia in respiratory diseases.
74. What is respiratory pulse and the condition?
75. Branches of facial artery.
76. Allen's and modified Allen's test.
77. Accessory muscles of inspiration and expiration.
78. Clinical correlation between uses of accessory muscle.
79. Conditions with altered respiratory pulse ratio.
80. Why thoracoabdominal breathing in females and abdominothoracic in males?
81. What type of breathing in meningitis?
82. Respiratory centers.

83. Pulsus paradoxus.
84. Beer–Lambert law.
85. Other principles of pulse oximetry.
86. Apical impulse—definition.

Index

Page numbers followed by *f* refer to figure and *t* refer to table.

A

Abdomen, acute 15
Accessory muscles 12
Acid-fast bacilli 82
   staining 82
Acquired immunodeficiency syndrome 42
Adenopathy 113*f*
Admission, criteria for 125
Aegophony sign 79
Allergic disorders 32
Allergy 18
   testing 83
American Thoracic Society 74
Amphoric breathing 72
Anatomic shunts 39
Anatomical principles 1
Angina 29
Angiotensin-converting enzyme 21, 33
Angle of Louis 1, 2
Anthropometry 37
Antinuclear antibody 85
Aortic arch 110
Aortic knuckle 110
Aortopulmonary window 110
Apical impulse 54
   position of 52
Apical region 55
Apneustic breathing 52
Appetite, loss of 31
Arterial blood gas 126
Arterial oxygen saturation, decreased 39
Asbestos bodies 82
Aspergilloma 24
Aspiration pneumonia 32, 33
Asthma 32
   acute severe 124
   history of 34
   life-threatening 124
   moderate exacerbation of 123
   near-fatal 124
   severe 126
Ataxic breathing 52
Auscultation, principles of 71
Axillary area 4
Axillary line, posterior 7

B

Bacteroides 24
Barrel chest 48
Bell tympany 80
Bilateral coarse miliary shadows 118*f*
Bilateral cystic lesions 120*f*
Biot's breathing 52
Blood
   gases 126
   pressure 38
   routine 81
   tests 89
Bony cage 100
Bony landmarks 104*f*

Branding scars 38
Breast
    implant 103*f*
    tissue, absence of 101*f*
Breath sound, normal 72, 73*f*
Breathing
    disorders, sleep-related 84
    tubular 71, 72
    types of 51
Breathlessness 18, 26
    severe 125
Bronchial arterial embolization 135
Bronchial asthma 82, 84
    acute exacerbation of 123
Bronchial breath 72
    sounds 72, 73*f*
Bronchiectasis 44, 120*f*
Bronchophony 79
Bronchopulmonary segments 11, 11*t*
Budesonide 130
Bulbar conjunctiva 39
Bullous emphysema 78

C

Carboxyhemoglobinemia 40
Carcinoembryonic antigen 85*t*
Cardiac dullness 69
Cardiophrenic angles 111*f*
Cardiothoracic ratio, causes of increased 111
Cardiothoracic surgery 81
Cardiovascular system 44
Cavernous breathing 72
Cellulitis 29
Central cyanosis 39, 40
    causes 39
Central pneumonia 80
Central tendon 14

Certain important tests 84*t*
Cervical rib, left 105*f*
Chest
    expansion, measurement of 57, 57*f*
    pain 18, 29
    shape of 47
    size of 47
    topography 3, 4*f*, 6*f*
    type of 47
Chest wall
    anterior 6*f*, 60*f*
    expansion 56*f*
    lateral 7*f*
    posterior 6*f*, 60*f*
    right 102*f*
    subcutaneous calcifications, left 102*f*
    symmetry 48
Chest X-ray 100*f*-102*f*, 105*f*, 106*f*, 111*f*-113*f*, 115*f*-120*f*, 126
    cardiac size in 110*f*
    interpretation 121
    lateral view 93*f*
    mediastinal compartments in 107*f*
    normal 104*f*
    over penetrated 98*f*
    reading of 89, 98
    standard posteroanterior view 92*f*
    systematic reading of 96, 97
    underpenetrated 99*f*
Cheyne–Stokes breathing 52
Chronic obstructive pulmonary disease, acute exacerbation of 130
Clavicular fracture 104
Clavicular percussion 65

Clubbing 38
  causes of 44
  differential 45
  unidigital 45
Cobbler's chest 48
Coin test 80
Common respiratory symptoms 18, 19
Compensatory emphysema 66
Constitutional symptoms 18, 30
Costal angle 16
Costochondritis 29
Costophrenic angles 111*f*
Cough 18, 19
  barking 20
  bovine 20
  brassy 20
  causes of 21*t*
  characteristics of 21*t*
  dry 20
  paroxysmal 20
  types of 20
  with expectoration 22
COVID-19, tests for 82
Cracked pot resonance 67
Crackles 75
  midinspiratory 76
  production of 75
Cricoid cartilage 1
Crura tendon 14
Curschmann's spirals 82
Cyanosis 38, 39
Cystic fibrosis 84
Cystic lesion, well-defined 119*f*
Cysts and cavities 115

D

D'espine sign 80
Dark lung fields 98*f*

Diabetes
  history of 34
  mellitus 32
Diagnose tension pneumothorax 133
Diagnostic skin tests 89
Diaphragm 13, 13*f*, 111
Differential cyanosis 40
  causes 40
Direct percussion 65
Distal phalangeal depth 43, 44*f*
Dysphagia 18, 30
Dyspnea 18, 26-28
  chronic 27
  grading of 27
  on exertion 28
  subacute 27

E

Ear, nose, and throat 81
Early inspiratory crackles 76
Ectopic endometrial tissue 33
Emphysema 48, 66, 120*f*
Empyema 44
Endemic hemoptysis 26
Eosinophils 81
Epilepsy, history of 34
Erythrocyte sedimentation rate 81
Expiration, muscles of 12

F

Fever 30
  types of 31
Fissure, horizontal 114
Fluticasone 130
Forced expiratory volume 123, 125
Formoterol 130

Foul-smelling sputum 24
Fusobacterium 24

G

Garland's triangle 70
Gastroesophageal reflux disease 21, 29
Gastrointestinal system 45
Grocco's triangle 70

H

Hacking dry cough 20
Hamman sign 78
Headache 18
Heart 108
Heart border
  percussion of
    left 69
    right 69
  right 108
Hematemesis 26*t*
Hemoglobin 39
  abnormality 40
Hemoptysis 18, 24, 25, 26*t*, 134
  assessment 135
  management of 135
  minimal 25
  moderate 25
  position 135
Hepatopulmonary syndrome 28
Herpes 29
Hilar enlargement, bilateral 113*f*
Hilum 17, 111
Hoover's sign 52
Human immunodeficiency virus 81, 118*f*
Hypertension 32
  history of 34
  treatment for 33
Hypertrophic pulmonary osteoarthropathy 43

I

Icterus 38, 39
Idiopathic pulmonary arterial hypertension 19
Immunological tests 84
Implantable cardioverter defibrillator 38
Infra-axillary area 4
Inspiration 58
Intensive care unit 91
Intercostal neuralgia 29
Interferon-gamma release assays 85
Interphalangeal depth 43, 44*f*
Interscapular area 4
Interstitial lung disease 21, 116*f*
Interstitial reticular densities, bilateral diffuse 116*f*
Ipratropium bromide 127, 130
  combination of 130

J

Jugular venous pulse 38, 46
  causes of increased 46

K

Kronig's isthmus 8, 66
Kussmaul breathing 52
Kyphosis 50*f*

L

Larynx, lower border of 1
Late inspiratory crackles 76
Left costophrenic angle 112*f*
Left upper lobe 9
  bronchus 11
Light-emitting diode 82
Lingula 11
Liquid bridge hypothesis 76

Liver
  dullness 69
  function testing 83
Lobe
  surface anatomy of 8
  upper 9, 10
Lordotic view 93
Lovibond's angle 42, 42*f*
Lower lobe
  left 9, 10
  pneumonia 115*f*
  right 9, 10, 115*f*
Lower respiratory tract 47, 85
Lung
  abscess 21, 44
  carcinoma 117*f*
  diseases, radiological patterns of 114, 115*t*
  fields 114
  left 8, 10*f*
  lobes 9*f*, 10*f*
  malignancy of 41
  markings, prominence of 99*f*
  secondaries 116*f*
  surface anatomy of 8
  tissue, wedge of 11
  volumes 115, 120*f*
Lymphadenopathy 38, 41
Lymphangioleiomyomatosis 19
Lymphocytes 81
Lymphomas 42

M

Marfan syndrome 48
Massive hemoptysis 25
Mastectomy, right 101*f*
Mastitis 29
Mediastinal crunch 78
Mediastinitis 29
Mediastinum 14, 15*f*, 104, 107
  inferior 14, 108
  lower 108
  superior 107
  upper 107
Menorrhagia 39
Metallic cough 20
Methemoglobinemia 40
Midaxillary line 7
Middle and lower regions 55
Monophonic wheeze 74
Muscular fibers 13
Myalgia 29
Myocardial infarction 29
Myotatic irritability 66

N

Nebulizer solutions available 130
Nodular densities, bilateral 116*f*
N-terminal pro-brain natriuretic peptide 85

O

Obstructive airway diseases 12
Obstructive pulmonary disease, chronic 19, 39
Oral cavity 47
Orthodeoxia 28
Orthopnea 28
Ortner's syndrome 29
Over penetrated film 97
Oxygen 126
  saturation 125

P

Pallor 38
Palpation 53, 85
Parasitic infestation 101*f*
Paratracheal stripes 106*f*

Parietal pleura 15
Paroxysmal nocturnal dyspnea 28
Patent ductus arteriosus 40
Peak expiratory flow 125
Pectus carinatum 48, 49*f*
Pectus excavatum 48*f*
Pedal edema 38, 45
Pedigree chart 32*f*
Peptostreptococcus 24
Percussion 61
    anterior 62, 62*f*
    cardinal rules of 63
    lateral 63
    note, types of 66
    posterior 63, 63*f*
Peripheral cyanosis 40, 41
    causes 40
Pigeon chest 48
Platypnea 28
Pleura 15
    sac 15
Pleural diseases 115
Pleural effusion 71, 112*f*
    right 94*f*, 121*f*
Pleural rub 77
Pleuritic pain 29
Pleurodesis 134
Pleximeter finger 64
    middle phalanx of 64*f*
Plexor finger 64*f*
Pneumomediastinum 78, 134
Pneumonia 21
Pneumothorax 66, 71
    left-sided 78
    small 93
Polymerase chain reaction 82
Polyphonic wheeze 75
Positive end-expiratory pressure 129
Post-tussive suction 79
Premenstrual pain 29
Primary ciliary dyskinetic syndromes 84
Principal muscles 12
Profile sign 44
Pseudoclubbing 45
Pseudohemoptysis 26
Pseudomonas infections 23
Pulled trachea syndrome 73
Pulmonary artery, left 110
Pulmonary edema 21
Pulmonary emergencies, management of 123
Pulmonary function testing 83
Pulmonary squeak 76
Pulmonary tuberculosis 85, 119*f*
Pulse 37
    oximetry 38, 125
Pursed lip breathing 52
Pyopneumothorax 68

R

Radial pulse
    left 38
    right 38
Rapid shallow breathing 52
Rectus abdominis 12
Renal function testing 83
Respiration
    abnormalities in 51
    muscles of 11
    types of muscles of 11
Respiratory diseases, symptoms of 19
Respiratory evaluation, common investigations in 81
Respiratory failure 136-138
    classification 136
Respiratory illness, history of 134

Respiratory movements 55
Respiratory rate 38
Respiratory system 44
   anatomy of 1
   diseases of 17
   examination of 37, 47
Retrosternal thyroid 20
Rhonchi 74
Rib 3
   cage 12
   erosions 29
   fracture of 29, 104
   fusion of 105*f*
Rifampicin 33
Right clavicle, bony mass in 106*f*
Right lateral decubitus film 94*f*
Right lung 8, 10*f*
   mass lesion 117*f*
Right middle lobe 9, 10, 115*f*
   bronchus 11
Right upper lobe 9, 10, 96*f*
   bronchiectasis 17
   bronchus 11
Roentgenography 89
Rule out artifacts 96

S

Salbutamol 130
Scalene muscles 12
Scapula, spine of 4
Scapular line 7
Schamroth's sign 43, 43*f*
Scoliosis 51*f*
Scratch sign 80
Serratia marcescens 26
Serum
   angiotensin-converting
      enzyme 85
   bilirubin 39
Shifting dullness 68
   percussion for 68

Shock 134
Shoulder, drooping of 50*f*
Skodaic resonance 67
Sleep
   disordered breathing 52
   disturbances 18, 30
Smoking index 32
Sneezing, rhinitis 18
Soft tissue 100
   bilateral 100*f*
   calcifications 101*f*
   density 103*f*
Solitary pulmonary nodule 89
Sounds
   added 74
   adventitious 74
Spinal abnormalities 49
Spinous process 16
Splenic dullness 70
Spurious hemoptysis 25
Sputum collection 82
Sputum malignant cytology 82
Squamous cell carcinoma 85
Sternal percussion 65
Sternocleidomastoid sign 52, 53*f*
Steroid therapy 127
Stony dull 67
Straight line dullness 68
Stress relaxation quadrupole
      hypothesis 75
Stridor 18, 30, 52
Succussion splash 78
Suprascapular area 4
Symptomatology 17

T

Tactile vocal fremitus 61
Tension pneumothorax 132
   causes 132
   examination 133
   possible complications 134

prognosis 134
symptoms 133
treatment 133
Thoracic cavity 12, 13
Thoracic movements 52
Thoracic vertebra 114
Tidal percussion 68
Tietze syndrome 29
Trachea 1, 104
   palpation of 54*f*
Tracheal descent 58
Tracheal tug 58
Trail's sign 52, 53*f*
Transversus abdominis 12
Trapped air increases, amount of 132
Traube's space 3, 70
Trepopnea 28
Tuberculous lymphadenopathy 41

U

Upper airway cough syndrome 24
Upper respiratory tract 1, 47, 85

V

Vena cava, superior 3
Ventilatory respiratory failure 137
Ventilatory support 129
Vertebral line 7
Vesicular breath sound 72
Virchow's node 42
Vital signs 37
Vocal fremitus 58, 60*f*
   examination 61*f*
Vocal resonance 77
Voice, hoarseness of 18, 29

W

Weight loss 31
   significant 31
Wheeze 18, 30, 74
   mechanisms of 74
Whispering pectoriloquy 79

X

Xiphisternum 14, 16

EU GSPR Authorised Reprsentative
Logos Europe, 9 rue Nicolas Poussin
1700, La Rochelle, France
Phone: +33 (0) 6 67 93 73 78
E-mail: contact@logoseurope.eu

www.ingramcontent.com/pod-product-compliance
Ingram Content Group UK Ltd.
Pitfield, Milton Keynes, MK11 3LW, UK
UKHW021827140426
5217IPUK00016B/1238